Handsome,

I love you!

Start eating right. No

more mayo, eggs or cheese!

Love You,

CODY

D0091992

YOU DON'T HAVE TO BE A
TREE-HUGGER
TO BE A VEGAN

Eating Healthy Is For Everyone

The *30 Days To Leave Your Blubber*™ Program

Dan Vishny

Printed in the U.S.A.

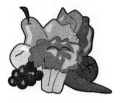

Copyright © 2005 by Dan Vishny
All rights reserved.

No part of this book may be reproduced in any form or by any electronic or mechanical means including information storage and retrieval systems, without permission in writing from the author, except by a reviewer, who may quote brief passages in a review.

Library of Congress Cataloging-in-Publication data is available.

ISBN 0-9772493-0-1

All information provided in this book, is presented for general informational purposes only. It should not be considered complete or exhaustive. It is not intended to be a substitute for the medical diagnosis, advice or treatment of physicians or other health care professionals. The information provided throughout this book should not be used for diagnosing or treating a medical problem, disease, or psychiatric problem or disorder. You should also not use the information in this book as a substitute for professional medical or psychiatric advice when deciding on any health-related regimen, including diet or exercise. Each individual should consult his or her own dietician and/or physician to design a diet that is appropriate in light of their own health condition and specific circumstances. In the event you use information from this book without your doctor's approval, you are prescribing for yourself, and the author assumes no responsibility.

This book is dedicated to you, the reader, and anyone that you care about. Opening and reading this book may lead you to a few more years of laughter and enjoyment with the ones you love, and give you enough time to use up your frequent flyer miles.

TABLE OF CONTENTS

"It's not the years in your life that count. It's the life in your years"
- *Abraham Lincoln* (1809-1865)

"Be careful about reading health books. You may die of a misprint."
- *Mark Twain* (1835-1910)

Introduction

How many more fad diets are going to be invented? What is the shelf life of a fad diet? They come and go with the tide. How about a diet that has been around for roughly four million years? How about a diet where all you do is listen to your mother—Mother Nature. At Mama Nature's Restaurant, the menu does not include food in a box, food that clogs your arteries, or food that comes with a pill to take so that you can digest it. Mama only serves natural, wholesome food—she knows what is best for you. By the way, she serves much more than tofu and sprouts.

This book is about reaching your natural health potential without sacrificing your love for eating. It shows a different point of view than the multitude of books out there regarding diet and health. The stereotype for a vegetarian/vegan is the Birkenstock-wearing, tree-hugging, animal rights activist. While protecting and preserving the environment and anti-cruelty to animals are important issues, they are not the focus of this book. Eating healthy does not have to be a political statement, it can be a personal health decision.

The usual pro-vegan reasons will be presented, as well as the opposing views. I have also included chapters on some interesting topics such as processed foods and food additives, genetically modified foods, how cheese is made, and organic vs. non-organic food. After you read the material, if you decide that you want to try a vegan diet, I offer an easy 30 day program. If you decide that you're not interested, that's cool too—at least you have increased your knowledge and will be able to understand what all the "hoopla" is about this vegan stuff.

Whether you want to lose weight or not, adhering to a vegan diet will eventually transform your body into the shape that nature intended. I can guarantee you this—you will look at food differently, you will learn something from the experience, and no physical harm will come to you. Your lifestyle does not have to change, but reading this book may change your life.

IT IS NEVER TOO LATE TO CHANGE YOUR HABITS AND IMPROVE YOUR HEALTH

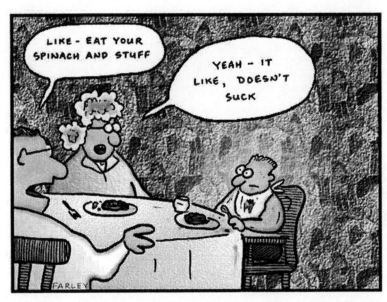

2010: The Beavis & Butthead generation grows up

Chapter 1

MY STORY AND
I'M STICKIN' TO IT

Breakfast: Cap'n Crunch® and milk

Lunch: bologna sandwich and milk

Afternoon Snack: candy bar or bag of chips

Dinner: meat, potatoes, and can of veggies

After Dinner Snack: ice cream or cookies

That is how I lived the first 18 or so years of my life. I grew up always a bit on the chunky side, had numerous yearly bouts with the flu, throat infections and colds. I never had any major health issues, but always carried a spare tire around my waist.

At around the age of 18, I started to become aware of my "unhealth". I simply did not feel healthy. I can't explain it exactly, I just felt yucky. Deep down, I knew that there was a better way. I started to eat less red meat and more chicken. The unfortunate trade-off was that I ate more dairy. I substituted frozen yogurt for ice cream—the word "yogurt" meant that it was better for you. I thought that was the answer.

After years of fooling myself, at around the age of 27, I decided to try a vegetarian diet. I remember the moment I told myself to go for it. I was in my car pulling into a Wendy's® parking lot to get my daily lunch of two grilled chicken sandwiches. I only ordered the grilled (not the fried) because that

4

was the healthy option—little did I know that the grilled chicken sandwich was injected with beef flavoring. I had been toying with the idea of trying a vegetarian diet. For some reason, I turned my car around, went home and made a peanut butter sandwich and drank a glass of milk.

I first cut out meat and fish, and after two weeks, I felt a little better. I had more energy, dropped a few pounds, but still nothing earth-shattering. I was still consuming a lot of dairy. One of my normal dinner meals consisted of half a loaf of French bread and a hunk of Gouda cheese. I loved cheese, I couldn't live without pizza. I promised not to get pepperoni, just give me mushroom and onion instead, I'll even get the extra thin crust, just don't take my pizza away.

Trying to be honest with myself I really did not feel that much healthier as a vegetarian. Reluctantly, I decided to take it a step further. I was nervous about this step. I didn't think I'd be able to stick to it. I figured I'd be knee deep in a deep dish pizza in a week. When I stopped eating dairy, what I discovered, was that my body seriously transformed. Within weeks, I lost more fat, and had even more energy. Within months, I completely lost my spare tire around my waist. After one year, I was back to my wrestling weight from high school. I did not get sick that entire year, not even a cold. This was the first time in my life that I actually felt healthy.

Since then, I have been on raw vegan diets and done numerous yearly fasts and cleanses—a topic for later discussion. The main point is that, after 12 years, I have never looked back. I can't look back, this is the way that my body was meant to eat. I don't really care how many years I live, I just want them to be fun-filled and healthy. To me, feeling healthy and alive is more important than a cheeseburger and a slice of pizza.

I used to always be on the unhealthy side of the fence, crossing over to the healthy side every so often. It didn't work. I discovered that it is better to do the opposite—live on the healthy side and splurge every now and then. Making the switch to the healthy side, in all honesty, was not difficult. If I could do it, anyone can. The hardest part was turning around in the Wendy's® parking lot—taking that first step.......

Each journey begins with a single step

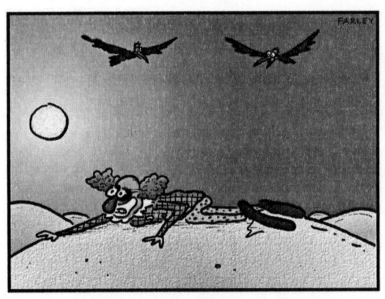

"Hey – Look! A Happy Meal!"

Chapter 2

 HEALTH, WELLNESS AND WHOLENESS

What do Plato, Benjamin Franklin, Gandhi, Leonardo DaVinci, Albert Einstein, Henry David Thoreau and Bob Marley all have in common? They all advocated a vegetarian diet.

> "In America today, poor diets are typically too high in calories and fats, and too low in fruits and vegetables, problems associated with certain chronic diseases and obesity."
> *-United States Department of Agriculture*
>
> "There is compelling evidence that a diet rich in fruits and vegetables can lower the risk of heart disease and stroke."
> *-Harvard School of Public Health*
>
> "I am living without fats, without meat, without fish, but am feeling quite well this way. It almost seems to me that man was not born to be a carnivore."
> *-Albert Einstein* (1879-1955)
>
> "I didn't fight my way to the top of the food chain to be a vegetarian."
> *-Unknown*

What is all the hoopla about this vegan thing? We've got liberal conservatives, conservative Republicans, and now vegan vegetarians—what's this all about? The answer is plain and simple—health. Is it the fountain of youth? No, not quite. Is it the fountain of health? Yes, absolutely.

8

Studies by independent, reputable organizations have shown that vegetarians/vegans are healthier and live longer than non-vegetarians. Most people are not surprised when they hear this. The usual reply goes something like this; "of course you live longer, you eat grass, you don't drink, you don't have fun, you're too busy out hugging trees, and protecting chickens." That is not true.

Being a vegan is not boring, it is not a sacrifice, and it does not have to be a political statement. You do not have to change your lifestyle or beliefs to be a vegan. The only requirements are to pay attention to what you eat and maintain a little discipline. It's really not that difficult.... and if you ever get hungry, you can just munch on your neighbor's lawn.

In the U.S., over 400,000 deaths a year are related to poor diet and physical inactivity. About 60 million American adults are obese; and 64% of adults between the ages of 20 and 74 are either overweight or obese. Overweight, obesity and physical inactivity are the major risk factors for chronic diseases such as diabetes, cardiovascular disease and cancer.

Can you remember the time in your life when you felt the healthiest? Can you remember how it felt? How different do you feel today? What is different? A couple of back pains? An achy knee? Becoming a vegan will not cure those ailments—that's just gravity up to its old tricks. But if you're tired of feeling blah inside and sick of looking at that spare tire around your waist, read on.

FOOD IS FUEL

Your body is a living machine. Compare it to an automobile. If you fill your auto's gas tank with polluted gas or the wrong gas, it will not run properly. The car will eventually break down, and you'll have to take the bus. Your body is no different.

Your body requires energy to process the food that you eat. The less energy that your body uses to process food, the more energy that it has for other stuff, like fighting disease. The more energy that your body uses to process food, the less energy your body has leftover. What happens to you after a big steak dinner, or a serving of Fettuccine Alfredo? You get tired and pray that there is something good on television. Your body gets zapped of its energy.

Imagine that your body is brand new and clean on the inside. Imagine that you have absolutely nothing in your digestive system. You just took the biggest dump in the history of mankind and your body has nothing left in the tank. Imagine how alive you feel. Now imagine feeding it an orange. It takes very little energy to turn that orange into fuel—it's enough fuel for hours. Your body is still full of energy. Now imagine eating a bacon egg muffin thingamajig—what's going to happen? Your energy is zapped and you just polluted your body with toxins. If you feed your body clean burning fuel, it will run better.

YOU ARE THE ONLY HEALTH EXPERT

One day the so-called "experts" say one thing, the next day, a new study comes out and they switch positions. You got laboratory studies, case-control studies, and randomized test trials. My advice is to throw away your health magazines, if they didn't have new reports and studies to publish, they wouldn't sell magazines. Further, turn off the evening news when they start to talk about the lady who eats dirt and lives to be 100 years old.

When it comes to your health, why not listen to the one person who you can trust, the one person who should tell you the truth—YOURSELF. When it comes to your body, you are the expert. Find out for yourself what the best diet is for you. If you don't feel right, or look right—then you're probably correct! Change it. Maybe becoming a vegan is the right alternative for you, maybe it's not. You will never know until you try. Don't be afraid to explore and to change—change is just growth in disguise.

In the end, you can't fool Mutha Nature, so why fight her? Work with her, not against her. Get your body back to its natural, undisturbed, clean state. Get your body into its natural form and you will feel better. Get your body in shape and your mind will follow.

> "Well-planned vegan and other types of vegetarian diets are appropriate for all stages of the life cycle, including during pregnancy, lactation, infancy, childhood, and adolescence."
> *-American Dietetic Association*

What are the different types of vegetarians?

- **Lacto-Ovo Vegetarian:** A person who does not eat meat, poultry, or fish, but eats dairy and egg products.
- **Ovo Vegetarian:** A person who does not eat meat, poultry, fish or dairy products, but eats egg products.
- **Lacto Vegetarian:** A person who does not eat meat, poultry, fish, or eggs, but eats dairy products.
- **Vegan:** A person who does not eat any animal products including meat, poultry, fish, eggs, or dairy.

In my opinion, the term "vegan" should be further divided into the following:

- **Orthodox Vegan:** A "strict" vegan who does not eat any animal products, or use any product derived from or tested on an animal. Further, if any harm or discomfort is inflicted on an animal in the process or procurement of a product, an orthodox vegan will not use it. Examples include leather, silk, wool, down and pearls.
- **Non-Orthodox Vegan:** A "not-so-strict" vegan who does not eat animal products, but uses products derived from animals. This person is strict in the dietary sense but not strict in the use of animal products.

The focus of this book is in regards to the non-orthodox vegan, your personal philosophy is your own business.

What about athletic performance?

Many studies have been conducted in regards to a vegetarian diet and its effect on athletic performance. They all pretty much say the same thing: it's not better or worse than a non-vegetarian diet. There are no differences in strength, fitness, or performance between vegetarian and non-vegetarian athletes. There are many vegan/vegetarian professional athletes: Carl Lewis, winner of nine Olympic Gold Medals; Martina Navratilova, champion tennis player; Dave Scott, six-time Ironman Champion, and Bill Pearl, former Mr. Universe, just to name a few.

Potential iron and zinc deficiencies are the two most common dietary deficiencies among any athletes, including vegetarian ones. Vegetarian athletes, and any athlete for that matter, should make sure to consume ample amounts of food containing iron and zinc, especially during times of heavy exercise.

Common Myths

Myth 1: You cannot obtain enough protein, calcium, vitamins and minerals from a vegan diet. *Studies show that a vegan diet provides adequate amounts of all the above.*

Myth 2: Tofu tastes like rubber. *I agree. Some people like it, some people don't.*

Myth 3: I'm going to starve on a vegan diet. *This isn't Jenny Vegan Craig. You can eat as much and as often as you want.*

THE AVERAGE AMERICAN EATS IN A LIFETIME

24 HOGS
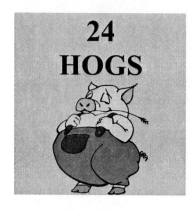

15 COWS
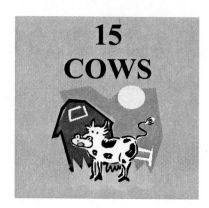

12 SHEEP
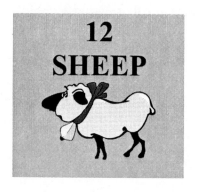

900 CHICKENS
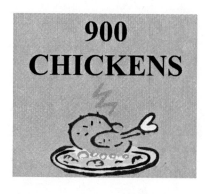

1000 lbs of CHEESE
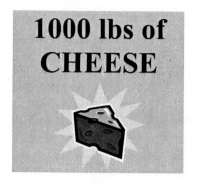

863 lbs of FISH
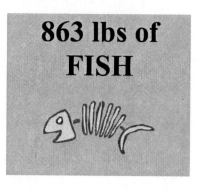

Chapter 3

CAN VEGANS EAT ANIMAL CRACKERS?
The Protein Question

"Protein requirements are readily met in children and adults eating a varied diet based on cereals and pulses."
-*World Health Organization*

"Plant protein can meet requirements when a variety of plant foods is consumed and energy needs are met."
-*American Dietetic Association*

"Cancer is most frequent among those branches of the human race where carnivorous habits prevail."
-*Scientific American 1892*

"If you ate pasta and antipasto, would you still be hungry?"
-*Unknown*

If there is one thing that everyone agrees on—the FDA, the AHA, the CIA, and my mother, it's that we all need protein in our diet. It is vital to our bodies' functioning. However, there is no consensus on where to get protein from. You know what the National Dairy Council is going to say. You know what the Cattle Ranchers Association is going to say. You know what Flo at Mel's Diner would say: "a cheese omelet, bacon, glass of milk, and kiss my grits."

Vegetables contain protein. In fact, all plant foods contain protein. Would you believe that a cup of broccoli has as much protein as three rib eye steaks? Not really, but it does contain as much protein as an egg (and you don't get the 215mg of cholesterol with the broccoli). Though you have to eat more than just broccoli, you can get enough protein from a vegan diet—I'm living proof.

How much protein do you need?

You need as much protein as your body tells you. The "experts" have never made up their minds as to how much protein we need to sustain a healthy body. Even if they came to a consensus, it wouldn't mean much, since everyone's body is different. Obtaining enough protein is usually not an issue, since most Americans consume 50 percent more daily protein than is required. The problem is not the quantity of protein, rather it is the quality.

If you want a generalized number, The Food and Nutrition Board, part of the National Academy of Sciences, says take your weight (in pounds) and multiply it by .36 – this is your daily recommended protein intake (in grams). Keep in mind this is an overstated, generalized guideline, not a strict rule. Counting grams of protein is not necessary, listening to your body (explained later) is what matters.

On the following page, I have included a table which shows values for some common foods. For an extensive list, go to *www.usda.gov*, where you can find nutritional values for just about everything (except circus peanuts).

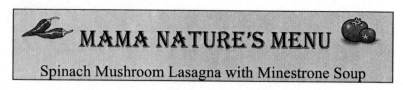

MAMA NATURE'S MENU

Spinach Mushroom Lasagna with Minestrone Soup

Table 1: How Much Protein Is In Certain Foods

Food Type	Serving Amount	Protein (grams)
Almonds	1 oz.	6.03
Bagel	1 bagel	8.72
Beans, pinto	1 cup	15.41
Beef, ground	3 oz.	21.73
Broccoli	1 cup	5.70
Butter	1 tbsp	0.12
Cheese, cheddar	1 oz.	7.06
Cheese, cream	1 tbsp	1.09
Cheeseburger	1 each	15.96
Chicken	1 leg	12.45
Chickpeas	1 cup	14.53
Collard greens	1 cup	4.01
Corn	1 cup	5.06
Couscous	1 cup	5.95
Doughnut	1 each	2.34
Egg, whole	1 each	5.54
Fish, cod	3 oz	19.51
Fish, salmon	3 oz.	16.81
Ham	2 slices	3.47
Ice Cream	½ cup	2.55
Lamb	little one	21.72
Lentils	1 cup	8.00
Lettuce, iceberg	I head	4.85
Lima beans	1 cup	14.66
Lobster	3 oz.	17.43
Milk	1 cup	8.26
Peanuts	2 tbsp	8.00
Peas	1 cup	5.23
Pepperoni pizza	1 slice	10.12
Potatoes	1 potato	5.00
Raisins	1 cup	4.45
Rice, Brown	1 cup	5.00
Soy milk	1 cup	10.98
Tempeh	1 cup	9.50
Tofu	¼ block	6.63
Turkey	3 oz	18.13
Veg Burger	1 patty	14.00
Yogurt, plain	8 oz	9.92
Yogurt, soy	8 oz.	8.00

Plant Protein vs. Animal Protein

Would you agree that a peanut butter sandwich is a healthier source of protein than a cheeseburger? If your sole diet consisted of cheeseburgers, what would happen to your body? If your sole diet consisted of peanut butter, what would happen to your body? It has been shown that the higher your intake of animal protein the higher your risk of cancers, heart disease, osteoporosis, and other health issues described below.

Does meat have more protein than vegetables? Yes, absolutely. However, in the Western world, we do not have a problem with getting enough protein, vegans or non-vegans alike. What we have a problem with is eating too much protein, and from the wrong sources.

Cancer:

Many forms of cancer, including colon, breast, prostate, and ovarian have been directly linked to meat consumption. The more meat that one consumes, the higher the risk. Eating meat cooked at high temperatures also increases the risk of cancers of the stomach, colon and rectum, since cancer causing substances (carcinogens) can form and bind to the surface of the food. In addition, the processes of curing or smoking meat may also produce harmful chemical substances which can adversely affect our health.

Fruits and vegetables contain antioxidants such as beta-carotene, and vitamins C & E which protect body cells against damage. The evidence is overwhelming that an abundant intake of fruits and vegetables can play an important role in reducing cancer risk.

Osteoporosis:

Consuming too much animal protein leaches calcium from the bones which can lead to osteoporosis or weakening of the bones (See Chapter 4).

Diabetes:

Vegetarians and vegans are less at risk from diabetes. Meat consumption is positively associated with diabetes in both males and females.

Gallstones:

Gallstones are formed when bile becomes saturated with cholesterol. The main risk factors are low fiber intake, high saturated fat intake, cholesterol intake and obesity. Non-vegetarians are twice as likely to develop gallstones.

Kidney Issues:

Consuming too much animal protein overworks the kidneys, which leads to their inability to filter waste from the body. Intake of animal protein has been directly associated with the risk of kidney stone formation. According to the American Dietetic Association, "a well-planned vegetarian diet may be useful in the prevention and treatment of kidney disease."

DID YOU KNOW?

Plant proteins contain the same 23 amino acids as animal proteins.

Cholesterol and Heart Disease:

The human liver produces all the cholesterol we need, so there is no dietary need for intake of cholesterol. Cholesterol is only found in foods of animal origin, such as meat, dairy, eggs, and fish. It is not found in any foods of plant origin, including nuts and legumes (and incidentally, french fries). In the U.S., heart disease is responsible for more than a half million deaths every year. For every 1 percent increase in the amount of cholesterol in your blood, there is a 2 percent increase in your risk of having a heart attack.

Table 2: Foods High in Cholesterol

Food	Serving Size	Cholesterol
Boiled Egg	1 egg	215 mg
Cream Cheese	3.5 oz	95 mg
Cheddar Cheese	3.5 oz	57 mg
Butter	3.5 oz	250 mg
Lamb	3.5 oz	70 mg
Beefsteak	3.5 oz	70 mg
Chicken	3.5 oz	60 mg
Kidney, beef	3.5 oz	375 mg
Liver, beef	3.5 oz	300 mg
Ice cream	3.5 oz	45 mg
Sponge Cake	3.5 oz	260 mg

DID YOU KNOW?

Shrimp and scallops contain more cholesterol than beef.

Table 3: Foods Low in Cholesterol

Food	Cholesterol
All vegetables	0 mg
All fruits	0 mg
All grains	0 mg
All nuts	0 mg
All seeds	0 mg
All vegetable oils	0 mg

There is no magic elixir or vitamin supplement which will counteract the negative effects of cholesterol. There is only one cure: reduce your intake. If you don't eat foods containing cholesterol, you won't have high cholesterol. The *British Medical Journal* published findings from a study concluding that vegans have a 57 percent reduced risk of death from heart disease. A vegan diet can not only lower the risks of getting heart disease, it can also halt and reverse the effects of it.

It is common knowledge that cholesterol is bad for you. Everyone knows it. We all watch our intake of it. It is so important that the government requires it to be listed on every nutritional label. So why do we consume foods that contain cholesterol? Your answer may be, because you can only obtain calcium from foods that also contain cholesterol. In the next chapter, I will explain that you can obtain an adequate amount of calcium from foods that do not contain cholesterol.

Is eating a steak every so often going to kill you? Probably not. Is eating an omelet with bacon once a week going to kill you? Again, probably not. However, overloading your body with animal protein will most likely lead to health issues later in life.

There are always exceptions to the rule. We have all heard stories of the person who was a chain-smoker for 50 years and never got lung cancer. However, we have heard more stories that did not turn out so well. It is the same with diet. You may be one of the lucky ones who can eat meat and cheese three times a day and never encounter health problems. But why take the chance? There are no proven health advantages to consuming a high protein diet, only disadvantages.

The percentage of animal protein in a typical Chinese diet is approximately 11 percent, whereas for Inuit Eskimos it is 90 percent. The Chinese are considered to be one of the healthiest cultures, as evidenced by the lower occurrences of disease when compared to other cultures. Eskimos have one of the shortest life expectancies of any culture. Is this due to their meat-based diet or the fact that they live in ice cubes and swim with polar bears?

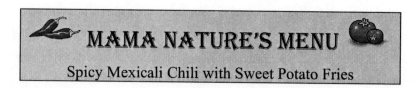
MAMA NATURE'S MENU
Spicy Mexicali Chili with Sweet Potato Fries

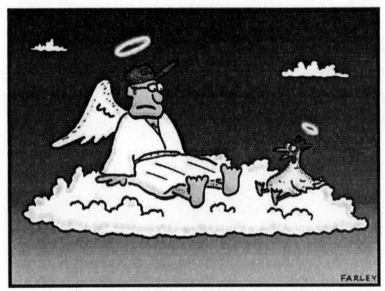

"I have to admit- I laughed when you
choked on that chicken bone"

Chapter 4

WHAT'S UP WITH THE
WHITE MUSTACHE?

> "A vegetarian, including vegan diet can meet current recommendations of **calcium**, protein, iron, zinc, vitamin D, riboflavin, vitamin B12, vitamin A, n-3 fatty acids, and iodine."
> *-American Dietetic Association*
>
> "Infants under the age of one should not drink whole cow's milk."
> *-American Academy of Pediatrics*
>
> "Save a cow. Eat a vegetarian."
> *-Unknown*

The human body needs calcium for building and maintaining bones and teeth, proper blood clotting, the transmission of nerve impulses, and the regulation of the heart's rhythm. Calcium is a vital nutrient. However, you do not need to nurse from a cow to get adequate calcium, you can obtain enough from plant sources. Calcium from plant sources does not come with risk factors such as osteoporosis, heart disease, cancer, and diabetes, described in the following paragraphs. Furthermore, it doesn't come in that gosh-dang milk carton that is always a pain in the butt to open.

The body obtains the calcium it needs in two ways. The first is by eating foods that contain calcium. The other is by borrowing it from our bones when calcium blood levels are low. If we borrow calcium from our bones and do not repay it to the bone bank, our bones eventually go bankrupt and break down—which is called "Osteoporosis". Osteoporosis or "porous bones" is the weakening of bones caused when bone destruction outweighs bone construction.

There are a number of factors that can reduce the risk of Osteoporosis:

Exercising regularly: This can be anything to keep the body moving, such as bicycling, weight training, swimming, yoga, and even simply walking. This does not include walking to the fridge to get another slice of cheesecake.

Getting enough Vitamin D: You can obtain enough Vitamin D either through diet or good old sunshine.

Getting enough Vitamin K: Vitamin K is found only in green leafy vegetables.

Avoiding too much Vitamin A: Preformed Vitamin A (not the beta carotene type) promotes bone loss.

Avoiding too much caffeine: Four cups of coffee or more can increase the risk.

Avoiding too much protein: Too much protein leaches calcium from your bones. Animal protein (dairy included) has been scientifically proven to cause more calcium leaching than vegetable protein sources.

Consuming enough calcium: Eat enough calcium so that you can pay back what you borrow from your bones.

Dairy intake does not lower the risk of osteoporosis and weak bones, and in many cases it increases the risk. Studies have shown that increased intake of dairy products is associated with a high risk of bone fracture and that there is no evidence that dairy or non-dairy sources of calcium protects the body from bone fracture.

Additional studies have shown that consumption of dairy products at a young age (around 20 years of age) leads to an increase in hip fractures at an older age (65 years and older). These and many other studies have discovered that the higher the intake of animal protein (meat and especially dairy sources), the higher the risk of weak bones. The reason seems to be that animal protein causes calcium to be leached from the bones.

Consuming dairy products that are high in saturated fat and cholesterol increase the risk of heart disease, whereas a vegan diet can prevent heart disease and also may reverse it. Consuming dairy products has also been linked to many types of cancer including colon, breast and prostate cancers and insulin-dependent diabetes (Type I or childhood-onset).

Lactose Intolerance

Lactose intolerance is the inability to digest milk sugar, and it causes symptoms such as gas, bloating, and abdominal pain. It is very common among many populations, affecting approximately 95 percent of Asian Americans, 74 percent of Native Americans, 70 percent of African Americans, 53 percent of Mexican Americans, and 15 percent of Caucasians. One study suggested that 75 percent of the population worldwide is thought to be lactose intolerant.

Health Concerns for Infants and Children

Dairy products also pose health risks for children and can lead to the development of chronic diseases such as obesity, diabetes, and early formation of atherosclerotic plaques that can lead to heart disease. The American Academy of Pediatrics recommends that infants below one year of age not be given whole cow's milk, as iron deficiency is more likely on a dairy-rich diet. Furthermore, it is not recommended that nursing mothers consume dairy, since one out of every five babies suffers from colic. Breastfeeding mothers can have colicky babies if the mothers are consuming cow's milk, since the cows' antibodies pass through the mother's bloodstream into her breast milk and to the baby.

How much calcium do we need? The current U.S. government recommendation for calcium intake is 1,000 mg/day for adults aged 19-50 and 1,200 for adults 50 and over. However, there is growing international evidence that these recommended calcium intakes are well overstated. For example, in countries where average calcium intake is 300 mg/day, such as India, Peru, and Japan, the occurrence of osteoporosis is low. Further, in the U.K., the recommended level for adults aged 19-50 is only 700 mg/day.

Where do vegans get their calcium? Calcium doesn't grow on trees? Well, actually it does, and it also grows in the ground.

> ### DID YOU KNOW?
>
> There are over 4,500 species of mammals in the world and only one species consumes milk after weaning.

Table 4: Good Plant Sources of Calcium

Vegetables	mg	Grains and Cereals	mg
Collard Greens,1 cup	357	TOTAL, ¾ cup	1104
Spinach, 1 cup	291	Corn Tortilla	120
Bok Choy, 1 cup	250	Oatmeal, 1 packet	105
Kale, 1 cup	179	Pita Bread	52
Okra, 1 cup	177	Wheat Flour, 1 cup	41

Nuts and Legumes	mg	Fruits	mg
Soybeans, 1 cup	261	Figs, 10 dried figs	269
White Beans, 1 cup	191	Raisins, 1 cup	73
Tofu, 1/4 block	163	Papaya, 1 whole	73
Pinto Beans, 1 cup	79	Dates, 1 cup	70
Almonds, 1 oz.	70	Orange, 1 whole	56
Tahini, 1 tbsp	64	Blackberries, 1 cup	46

DID YOU KNOW?

3/4 of a cup of collard greens has more calcium than a cup of milk.

As I promised, I'm not going to sling too much veggie gospel without presenting the other point of view. Here is some pro-dairy information from the website *www.whymilk.com.*

Table 5: Milk is Fuel for Athletes[1]

Low fat or fat-free milk is an ideal drink to help fuel physical activity...here are some good reasons why:

Strengthens Bones, Promotes Healthy Weight - Milk not only helps build bone mass and maintains bone density, but recent studies have also shown that teenagers who drink milk tend to be leaner than those who don't.

Maintains Lean Body Mass - The protein in milk contains all of the essential amino acids for building or maintaining your lean body mass. Three glasses of milk provides about half the protein you need each day.

The Ultimate Sports Recovery Drink - When it comes to refueling after exercise, new research suggests chocolate milk can be just as effective, if not more, than traditional sports drinks. Researchers found it helps athletes recover from an intense workout and is an effective exercise recovery drink to refuel exhausted muscles - allowing for future enhanced performance.

Provides Essential Electrolytes - Potassium is crucial to regulate the balance of fluids in the body and also is needed for muscle activity and contractions. Cup for cup, milk has 10 times more potassium than the leading sports drink.

Gets You Energized - Milk contains B-vitamins such as B-12, niacin and riboflavin, which are necessary to convert food to energy for exercising muscles. One glass of milk also provides 20 percent of the phosphorus you need each day, which helps strengthen bones and generates energy in your body's cells.

Keeps You Hydrated - Milk is 90 percent water so it can help provide fluid to keep you hydrated.

---

[1] Reprinted with permission from *www.whymilk.com,* the online educational resource for consumers from MilkPep, (Milk Processors Education Program), funded by America's Milk Processors. *"Fuel for Athletes".*

For additional pro-dairy information, I have included some research which was submitted to the U.S. Department of Health and Human Services in March, 2004 (by the National Dairy Council®).

A New Zealand study concluded that boys and girls between the ages of 3 and 13 who avoid drinking cow's milk are more prone to bone fracture. This study also said fractures are to some degree a matter of chance because bones rarely break spontaneously and a limitation on the study was its small sample size (30 girls and 20 boys).

Another study concerning adolescent females concluded that there is a positive influence of calcium supplementation and intake of dairy products on bone mineral density of the hip and forearm. This study was supported by grants from the USDA and the National Dairy Council.

Finally, another study determined that women with low milk intake during childhood and adolescence have less bone mass in adulthood and greater risk of fracture. There was a large sample of subjects in this study, but the authors noted that conclusions from this study are limited due to the fact that milk intake during childhood was ascertained by recall and other calcium sources, such as plant sources were not measured.

OK, enough with the research already. You'll find research for and research against consumption of dairy. There's even a study that shows a positive relationship between intake of cola beverages and bone fracture. Again, you make the decision if it's right for you. Here are my final thoughts on the matter....

Table 6: History of Man

HUMAN SPECIES	TIME PERIOD
Ardipithicus ramidus	5 to 4 million years ago
Australopithecus anamensis	4.2 to 3.9 million years ago
Australopithecus afarensis	4 to 2.7 million years ago
Australopithecus africanus	3 to 2 million years ago
Australopithecus robustus	2.2 to 1.6 million years ago
Homo habilis	2.2 to 1.6 million years ago
Homo erectus	2.0 to 0.4 million years ago
Homo sapiens archaic	400 to 200 thousand years ago
Homo sapiens neandertalensis	200 to 30 thousand years ago
Homo sapiens (us humans)	200 thousand years ago to now
Homo milkus the cow utterus	**4 thousand years ago to now**

The point of the above table is that cows have been domesticated for only 4,000 years. On an evolutionary timeline, that is miniscule. Even if our bodies have evolved over 2 million years in order to eat and process meat, our bodies have simply not had enough time to evolve to efficiently process another animal's milk. Mother's milk was made by mother nature for baby boys and girls. Cow's milk was made for baby cows, who grow 4 times faster than baby boys and girls. It is an entirely different substance. Maybe that's the reason that 75 percent of the world's population is lactose intolerant, and that we have so many health problems associated with dairy consumption. Our bodies simply don't like it.

Milk and dairy products are not necessary in the diet and can, in fact, be harmful to your health. Dairy products are not the best source of calcium as they promote calcium losses at the same time as increasing calcium intake.

31

Before we domesticated cows, we obtained all the calcium that we needed from plant sources. The reasons not to consume dairy: osteoporosis, heart disease, cancer, and diabetes. The reason to drink milk: the white mustache. Yes, milk is loaded with calcium, but it's also loaded with fat and cholesterol. The FDA says it, Ivy League schools say it, but yet they won't commit to saying dairy is bad for you. The one point that is not disputed is the fact that you can get enough calcium from non-dairy sources.

But you like the taste of dairy, I know, I used to like dairy too. But, you know deep down, that it may be bad for you. I used to like doing shots of tequila until 2 a.m., but I knew deep down it was bad for me—especially when I fell down the stairs. I used to like going to Vegas with my paycheck, but I knew it was bad for me when I came home with an Elvis keychain and an empty wallet.

You will get over it. It is not that hard. Trust me.

But I can't live without my cheese...

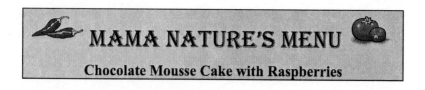

MAMA NATURE'S MENU

Chocolate Mousse Cake with Raspberries

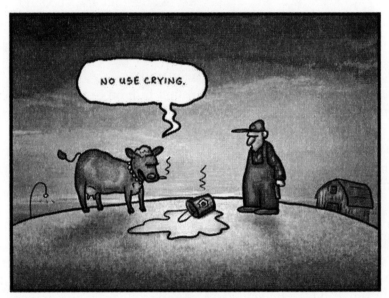

Milk Noir

Chapter 5

 ## IS IT EASY
BEING CHEESY?

> "Cheese, wine and a friend must be old to be good."
> -*Cuban Proverb*
>
> "The early bird may get the worm, but the second mouse gets the cheese."
> -*Unknown*

Legend has it that cheese was discovered by an Arab nomad who filled a saddlebag with milk to sustain him on his journey across the desert. After several hours of riding in the hot sun, he opened up the bag and discovered that the milk had separated into a watery liquid and solid white lumps (curds and whey). Instead of being able to enjoy his bowl of Fruit Loops®, the man had to settle for a grilled cheese sandwich.

Here is an abbreviated overview of how milk is actually turned into cheese: First, milk is pasteurized, which is simply heating it to destroy any harmful bacteria. Starter cultures (good bacteria) are added to the warm milk which changes a small amount of the milk sugar into lactic acid. This acidifies the milk and prepares it for the next stage—coagulation. Rennet, usually an extract from the fourth stomach of lambs and calves (cows and sheep have four stomachs), is then added to the milk and a curd is produced.

Curd grains fall to the bottom of the cheese vat, the left-over liquid (whey) is drained off, dehydrated and packaged in a can and called "protein powder." The curd grains that remain, bind together to form large slabs. The slabs are then milled, and salt is added to provide flavor and help preserve the cheese. The slabs are pressed and packed in various sized containers for maturing.

Cheese is allowed to "ripen", "age", "mature" or "mold" for various periods of time. During this time, bacteria continues to grow in the cheese, which changes its composition and more importantly, its flavor. Sometimes an additional microbe is added to a cheese. Blue veined cheeses are given a Penicillium spore which creates their aroma and flavor. Cheeses such as Camembert and Brie have their surfaces treated with a different type of Penicillium spore which creates a white mold.

RENNET: Why some cheeses are not vegetarian

Milk is coagulated by the use of certain plants or by extracting the enzyme "rennet" from the fourth stomach of calves. Records for the making of rennet go back to the 16th century. The cheese maker would slaughter a milk-fed calf, remove and wash the fourth stomach carefully, and hang it out to dry. The dried pieces of the stomach (called "vell") were added directly to the milk, and at later times vell extracts in salt solution were used.

Another form of rennet is called vegetable rennet which is derived from certain strains of fungi and bacteria. Today, this type of rennet is becoming popular, reflecting a move towards the manufacture of vegetarian cheese.

To summarize, cheese is just moldy milk. But, it tastes good on pizza and goes well with a Cabernet—I remember well. How do you replace the taste of cheese as a vegan? There are some very good soy cheeses and vegan cream cheeses, but they're not the real deal. The goal is to eat what nature intended, which in my opinion is not another animal's milk gone bad. So, you move on from cheese. It's like anything—you miss it less as time goes on. By the way, you can still enjoy pizza without cheese, and mushroom ravioli goes great with a Cabernet. Try cutting cheese out of your diet and see if your body likes the results. If the taste of cheese outweighs the results, then you go back to eating it.

What came first, the vegan or the egg?

> "Ham and eggs: a day's work for a chicken, a lifetime commitment for a pig."
> - *Unknown*

What are eggs? Are they meat, dairy or something else? If an egg was fertilized, it would be a chick and therefore would be considered meat (poultry). However, 99 percent or more of the eggs sold today are not fertilized. Some people define dairy products as only milk and milk byproducts, while others include eggs.

Regardless of what food category eggs fit into, they are not a healthy source of nutrition. One egg contains 4.5 grams of fat and 215 milligrams of cholesterol. The American Heart Association no longer makes a recommendation on how many eggs one is "allowed" to eat in a week; it used to be 3 to 4. However, they do recommend that egg yolks are limited to two per week for those at high risk or who already have heart disease.

Salmonella is another concern with egg consumption. According to the Center for Disease Control, every year, approximately 40,000 cases of salmonellosis are reported in the United States. Because many milder cases are not diagnosed or reported, the actual number of infections may be thirty or more times greater. Contamination usually occurs from eating mishandled or undercooked beef, poultry, or eggs.

The chances are not likely that you will get salmonella from eating eggs, especially if they are cooked and handled properly. Most studies show that eating eggs increases your cholesterol and hence your risk of heart disease. However, other studies show that moderate consumption of eggs does not increase your cholesterol. What is moderate? And are they counting the bacon and buttered toast that usually accompanies an egg breakfast?

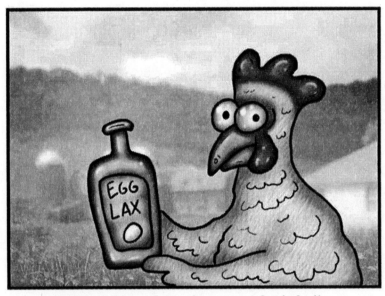

When chickens have that not so fresh feeling

Chapter 6

 **What was on the menu
200,000 years ago?
A Banana or a T-Bone?**

"Most of mankind for most of human history has lived on vegetarian or near-vegetarian diets."
- American Dietetic Association

"Man's structure, external and internal, compared with that of the other animals, shows that fruit and vegetables constitute his natural food."
-Karl von Linne (1707-1778), founder of taxonomy

"If we aren't supposed to eat animals, then why are they made of meat?"
-Unknown

What are we supposed to eat according to the laws of nature? This is an issue that has received much debate in the scientific community, more so than the debate over if Mickey is a mouse, and Pluto is a dog, then what the hell is Goofy?

Definitions
Carnivore: only eats animals
Herbivore: only eats plants
Omnivore: eats both plants and animals

Where do we fit into the above categories? Cats are carnivores, horses are herbivores and bears are omnivores. What are humans? The typical pro-vegetarian argument goes something like this:

Body design: The human body is not fit to run fast enough to catch prey as are carnivorous animals. Try tracking down a rabbit, chicken or pig; it's not natural. Furthermore, humans do not possess sharp claws which help in enabling carnivores to capture and kill prey.

Teeth and Mouth Structure: Our teeth and mouth structure are not designed to eat meat. We do not have powerful jaws and canine teeth to pierce and tear through flesh. Humans possess molars, which are designed for crushing and grinding seeds and vegetables, whereas carnivores possess canines.

Digestion: Carnivores have much shorter digestive tracts, 3-6 times their body length, than do humans which can be up to 11 times the length of a body. Carnivores do not chew their food, rather they tear it off in chunks and swallow it whole. Humans chew their food and possess an enzyme called "ptyalin" in saliva which aids in the digestion of food.

Natural Instincts: Most humans do not hunt or kill their meat, as all carnivores do in nature. Humans usually have to cook their meat and can rarely palate raw meat, which is the only way it is "served" in nature.

The typical pro carnivore/omnivore argument goes something like this:

Vitamins and Minerals: Humans require vitamin B12 for proper nutrition which can mainly be found in animal foods. Plant foods available in evolutionary times were poor in zinc and iron. The nutritional requirements for these minerals came from animal food sources.

Archaeological Evidence and Evolution: There is archaeological evidence, such as stone meat-cutting tools and animal bones, that prove humans were consuming meat as long as 2 million years ago. Humans could not have developed a larger brain unless we consumed meat, including insects. Cooking food might have made digestion less "expensive" in metabolic terms, thereby freeing up energy for increases in brain size.

Chimps Eat Meat and Gorillas eat Insects: Our closest living relatives eat meat and insects as part of their diet. Jane Goodall discovered that certain groups of chimps do eat meat when the opportunity arises, although it does not make up more than 2 percent of their overall diet. Gorillas, who are considered vegetarian by most standards, do (by accident or on purpose) consume insects on vegetation. Even though animal sources of protein are small compared to the overall diet, they still consume it and therefore, are omnivores.

Teeth and claws: Humans do not possess claws or sharp teeth because we have used technology, such as stone tools, silverware and the good old-fashioned meat grinder to serve the same function as claws and sharp teeth.

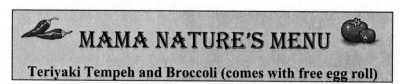

MAMA NATURE'S MENU

Teriyaki Tempeh and Broccoli (comes with free egg roll)

The Aquatic Ape Theory

Not that this is a science book, but this obscure yet interesting theory regarding human evolution is too cool to leave out. It states that many human physical characteristics can be explained by a semi-aquatic stage that our ancestors underwent in the past. It says that human ancestors may have lived and evolved on a flooded, semi-aquatic habitat, such as a mangrove. A brief overview of the evidence supporting this theory follows:

Human Hairlessness: All non-human mammals which have lost all or most of their fur are either swimmers like whales, dolphins, and walruses, or wallowers like hippopotamuses and pigs. A coat of fur may provide the best insulation for land mammals while the best insulation in water is not fur, but a layer of fat. There are two kinds of animals which tend to acquire large deposits of fat, hibernating ones and aquatic ones. While some of us lucky ones hibernate in the winter (to Florida or the south of France), humans as a general rule are not hibernating animals.

Bipedalism & Mating: Other than humans, two primates when on the ground stand and walk on two feet. One, the proboscis monkey, lives in the mangrove swamps of Borneo. The other is the bonobo or pygmy chimpanzee; its habitat includes a large tract of seasonally flooded forest. Bonobos often mate face-to-face as humans do; in our case it is explained as a consequence of bipedalism (walking on two legs). This mode of mating is rare among land animals, but which we share with a wide range of aquatic mammals such as dolphins, beavers and sea otters.

Breathing: Voluntary breath control appears to be an aquatic adaptation because, apart from ourselves, it is found only in aquatic mammals like seals and dolphins. When they decide how deep they are going to dive, they can estimate how much air they need to inhale.

What does this have to do with price of tofu in China? I'm not sure, but it's interesting. Actually, if the Aquatic Ape Theory has some validity, then these apes may have been the first fishermen. If humans had a semi-aquatic existence, they could have supplemented their plant-based diets with fish and Oysters Rockefeller.

There are still people today who live a life dependent on and in the water, such as the *Salon* of Myanmar (otherwise known as "Burma"). They are experts in swimming and diving. They are able to dive down to 60 feet and stay underwater for many minutes without using an oxygen tank. The *Salon* harvest marine products such as sea shells, oysters, mollusks, seaweeds, and pearls.

Discussion and Conclusion:

Before we discovered fire (approximately 200,000 years ago), I think you'd have a hard time telling humans and chimps apart. In my opinion, the human diet would have consisted of mainly fruits and vegetables and maybe the occasional trip to Ye Olde Termite Shoppe. Some chimps do hunt for and eat raw meat, but scientists state that many of these chimps do not live as long as a result of their meat eating—same as humans.

Ask yourself, could you eat raw meat? I'm not talking steak tartar at The Ritz. If someone places a platter of raw bush pig, a bowl of termites, and a bowl of strawberries in front of you, what are you reaching for? I'm having strawberry soufflé.

I have a difficult time envisioning ancient humans ripping apart a rodent, a deer, or a pig and eating the meat raw; they didn't have ketchup in the cupboard to hide the taste. Regardless, I do not think that our bodies were equipped for that kind of diet. But, some insects every now and then, or an occasional sushi platter?

If humans evolved from insectivores, why wouldn't they continue to eat insects? Or if we evolved from aquatic apes, why not throw in some California rolls when the tide was right? I wasn't there dressed in animal skins chasing bush pigs, so I can't say for sure what we ate.

If we weren't meant to eat meat, then why do we do it? That is a great question. On the other side, if our bodies were built for a heavy carnivorous diet, then why do we have so many diseases and disorders that are directly related to meat consumption. Who knows what the answer is? The important question remains, what is the healthiest, natural diet?

The most significant topic regarding this point is that all the discussion out there centers around are humans carnivores, omnivores or herbivores, not cow milkers. That is because dairy has not been a part of the human diet until recently, approximately 4,000 years ago. Further, there is nothing to compare us to in this regard, since we are the only species in the history of life to drink another animal's milk.

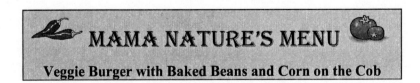

MAMA NATURE'S MENU
Veggie Burger with Baked Beans and Corn on the Cob

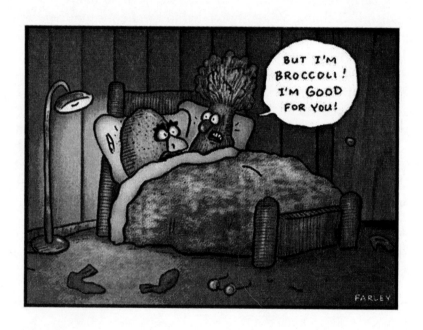

Chapter 7

 GONE FISHIN'?

> "Nearly all fish and shellfish contain traces of mercury."
> – *U.S. Dept. of Health & Human Services*
>
> "Almost every state has waters that are contaminated by industrial chemicals or other toxic substances."
> – *Field and Stream*
>
> "Recent findings indicate that susceptible populations continue to be exposed to PCBs via fish and wildlife consumption."
> – *Environmental Protection Agency*
>
> "Fish, to taste right, must swim three times: in water, in butter, and in wine."
> –*Unknown*

A fat fish- no way!

Fish are not always the low fat alternative to meat. Many fish, such as catfish, swordfish, shark, and sea trout, contain almost 33 percent fat, while salmon and orange roughy contain over 50 percent. Shrimp and prawns contain double the amount of cholesterol than beef, and a three ounce serving of salmon, contains the same as in a comparable serving of a T-bone steak. However, not all fish are created equal. There are many types of fish that have a lean fat content (See Appendix 2).

Some fish need to take a bath

Some fish are loaded with mercury, lead, and pollutants like PCB, DDT and dioxins. These chemicals have been linked to kidney damage, cancers, nervous disorders, impaired mental development, fetal damage, and many other health problems. The general rule is the higher up the food chain, the higher level of pollutants in the fish, and the "dirtier" the fish. Shellfish are extremely dirty due to their filter feeding method of eating.

Mercury rising

Mercury makes its way into the environment mainly through industrial pollution. Rain and snow washes it into waterways, where it is eaten by microorganisms, which are in turn eaten by fish, which are in turn caught by Fisherman Fred who sells it to your local grocery store. Nearly all fish contain traces of mercury. Eating fish contaminated with mercury can cause serious brain and nervous system damage—same as watching too many 80's sitcoms.

In the U.S., mercury levels in the environment have been increasing at an average rate of 1.5 percent each year since 1970. Forty-five states have fish consumption advisories. The Food and Drug Administration (FDA) and the Environmental Protection Agency (EPA) have advised that young children, women who are trying to become pregnant, women who are pregnant, or nursing to avoid certain types of fish that have high levels of mercury such as shark, swordfish, king mackerel, or tilefish (golden bass or golden snapper).

Additional research seems to indicate that people who consume fish such as tuna, swordfish, halibut, ahi, and sea bass have dangerously high levels of mercury in their blood. That is not to say that all fish have high levels of mercury. Fish that are usually low in mercury include shrimp, canned light tuna (not albacore), salmon, pollock and catfish.

If you want to see what the EPA recommended allowable intake is for a particular fish, check out the mercury calculator available at *www.gotmercury.com*. You put in your weight, the type of fish, and it tells you what the EPA limit on exposure is.

PCBs (Polychlorinated Biphenyls)

PCBs are man-made carcinogenic (cancer-causing) chemicals which have been banned for many years. However, testing has shown that the problem of PCB-contaminated fish is still widespread. As of 2003, more than two million lake acres and 130,000 river miles were covered by some type of PCB advisory.

According to the EPA:

"Recent findings indicate that susceptible populations (e.g., certain ethnic groups, sport anglers, the elderly, pregnant women, children, fetuses, and nursing infants) continue to be exposed to PCBs via fish and wildlife consumption. Human health studies indicate that: 1) reproductive function may be disrupted by exposure; 2) neurobehavioral and developmental deficits occur in newborns and continue through school-aged children who had in utero exposure to PCBs; 3) other systemic effects (e.g., self-reported liver disease and diabetes, and effects on the thyroid and immune systems) are associated with elevated serum levels of PCBs; and 4) increased cancer risks, are associated with PCB exposures."

DID YOU KNOW?

Salmon contains more cholesterol than a double cheeseburger.

Food poisoning risk

Seafood is the number one cause of food poisoning in the United States. The risk of food poisoning from eating fish and seafood is far greater than that from eating beef, pork or poultry. As much as 10 percent of raw shellfish are infected with organisms that can cause hepatitis, salmonella poisoning or cholera.

The Center for Disease Control in the U.S. reports an average of 325,000 food poisonings annually from contaminated seafood. This number represents only the reported findings, the actual number may be significantly higher.

Farm fresh fish?

Farmed salmon have significantly higher levels of toxic contaminants than salmon from the wild. Contamination by PCBs, dioxins and pesticides is on average 10 times higher in farmed salmon than in their wild relatives.

In the wild, salmon get that rich, pink color by consuming pink krill, but farmed fish are given a synthetic pigment called canthaxanthin in their food. Without it, their flesh would be an unappetizing, pale grey.

Omega-3 is not a star in the constellation of Veggus

The usual recommendations for eating fish are that they are lower in fat than other meats and it helps prevent heart disease and stroke because it contains the omega-3 fat. Omega-3 fatty acids benefit the hearts of healthy people, and those at high risk of or who have heart disease. However, many fish are not lower in fat than a lean cut of beef or chicken, and one can obtain just as much, if not more omega-3 from soybeans, canola and flaxseed oils.

Healthy Alternative to Meat?

I always thought that eating fish was a healthy alternative to eating meat. It is so embedded in my way of thinking, that even after doing the above research, I still have a difficult time believing that eating fish is not healthy, or at the very least, healthier than eating meat. The aspect of fish that is most bothersome to me is how dirty they are. They are basically toxin sponges—absorbing all the garbage that we dump into the waterways.

All the major health organizations say to eat fish, but not too much of it, especially if you are pregnant or a young child. If it's not good enough for a child, then it's not good enough for me. Furthermore, the "unsafe to eat" fish make the list after we have eaten it for awhile. There are probably more types of fish that will be added to this "unsafe to eat" list in the future. Lastly, if pollutant levels are on the rise, then it logically follows that the levels of toxins in fish can only get worse over time.

But to be honest, no matter how hard you try, you cannot add enough Hollandaise sauce to tofu to make it taste like Lobster Florentine. However, don't worry, there are many decadent meals that you will discover—and they don't come with a side order of salmonella, mercury, or chemicals whose names you can't pronounce.

If we could be guaranteed that we are getting a fresh, uncontaminated, low-fat fish, then it wouldn't be that bad—but where do you get that? Do you have to catch it yourself in the un-chartered waters of Alaska? How could you be sure that the fish didn't spend the last three years in Lake Sludgedump? Maybe it is better to err on the safe side, and not eat fish, or make it a once in a while meal, not a mainstay of your diet. Fish and seafood are not a necessary source of nutrition.

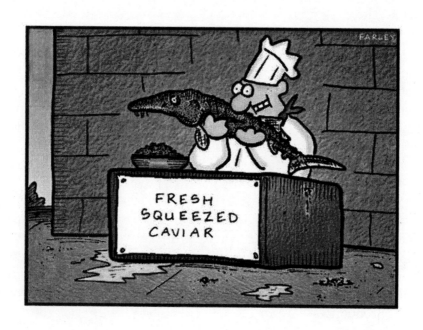

Chapter 8

WHAT ABOUT
HAPPY HOUR?

> "Beer is proof that God loves us and wants us to be happy."
> -*Benjamin Franklin* (1706 – 1790)

Can you go to happy hour with your friends? Are you allowed to have a cocktail before dinner? What about drinking a forty ounce out of a paper bag? The choice is yours. However, for your information, some producers use animal products in the "fining" or clarifying process of beer and wine production.

Finings are used to clarify beer or wine by binding loose materials and sinking to the bottom. These fining agents are removed from the beer/wine via filtration but no guarantee is made by manufacturers that there is no residue in the final product. Are trace amounts of this or that going to harm your health? Probably not, unless they're plutonium. It's up to you to decide how strict your diet and philosophy is.

Beer, Cerveza, Brew

Generally, cask-conditioned beers are fined using isinglass, which is derived from the swim bladders of certain tropical fish, usually sturgeon. On the other hand, keg, canned, and some bottled beers are usually fined without the use of this animal substance. Again, these fining agents are removed during filtration, but there is no guarantee that there is no residue.

Wine, Vino, Bubbly

Finings used in the production of wine include isinglass, gelatin, egg albumen, modified casein, and chitin. Vegan alternatives include bentonite, kieselguhr, kaolin and silica gel. The majority of organic wineries do not use animal derived finings. Winemakers in Burgundy, France commonly utilize egg whites in the production of wines above $15 a bottle or wines which are expected to age. The most popular substance used in domestically-produced white wines is bentonite. The generally accepted view is that the fining agents are removed before the wine is bottled.

The Hard Stuff: "Spirits" or "Hard Alcohol"

Most spirits are produced without any animal products, with the possible exception of some imported vodkas which may have been passed through a bone charcoal filter.

What's the Story with Sulfites in Wine?

All wines contain sulfites since they are a natural byproduct of fermentation. Most producers add additional sulfites to inhibit the growth of bacteria and to preserve the color in wine. Though most people do not have a health issue with sulfites, they are a serious hazard to some people, especially asthmatics, who are sensitive to these substances. In the U.S., all "organic wine" must be made without added sulfites.

It is generally accepted in the scientific community that sulfites do not cause headaches. However, drinking too much MD 20/20 out of a paper bag does usually lead to an increase in headaches.

Summary:

You make the call. The fining agents are supposed to be filtered out of the final product, but you can never be 100 percent certain. If you drink some microscopic amount of isinglass, is it going to kill you? Probably not. What may kill you is if you drink too much and fall down the stairs. I say, if you want to drink, then drink. It is more important to focus on the bigger picture and not get hung up on the technicalities. Asking a waiter at a restaurant to check if the marinara sauce is made with chicken stock is acceptable, but asking a hostess at a dinner party if the Cabernet Franc is filtered with the swim bladder of a Chinese sturgeon, is questionable.

The Vegetarian Network of Victoria has an excellent list of vegan friendly alcoholic beverages. To check it out visit *www.vnv.org.au/alcoholbyname*.

DID YOU KNOW?

Ox blood is still used as a wine clarifier in some Mediterranean countries.

Is Sugar Vegan?

Approximately half of the sugar in the U.S. is cane sugar, the other half is beet sugar. Beet sugar is vegan, cane sugar is questionable. During the refining process, cane sugar is filtered through charcoal, which has a 50/50 chance of being made from animal bones. The charcoal does not remain in the sugar itself, but it is used as a filter. Therefore, some people consider it to not be vegan.

You have probably heard of all the negative consequences of consuming too much sugar: tooth decay and diabetes to name a few. My main concern with refined sugar is that it is so highly processed, that by the time it reaches the sugar packet, all the nutrients have been zapped from it. Refined sugar passes through carbon filters, triple effect evaporators, pressure filters, vacuum pans, centrifugals, dryers, and conditioning silos.

There are many alternatives to refined sugar: turbinado, beet sugar, succanat, date sugar, fructose, barley malt, rice syrup, corn syrup, molasses, and maple syrup. Pure maple syrup is simply boiled tree sap and is a great replacement for refined sugar. It works well in coffee, iced tea, lemonade, and of course on pancakes (see recipe in Appendix 1).

What about Honey?

The Old Testament refers to the holy land as the "land of milk and honey". Honey has been found in the tombs of ancient Egypt. In ancient times honey was so valuable it was even used as currency—do we have a sweet tooth or what?

The National Honey Board will tell you that honey is good for you; the darker the honey, the higher the antioxidant content. Some people say that honey heals wounds, aids digestion, guards against ulcers, fights allergies, and smoothes the skin.

54

In the strict sense, it is not vegan. Bees are insects and insects are animals. Therefore, honey is an animal derived product. It is basically "milking" a bee. Is pure honey bad for your health? Probably not, it's just unrefined sugar.

In Conclusion or Collusion:

I probably eat too much sugar, I can't help it. I like maple syrup in my coffee and on my pancakes. I stay away from refined sugar, unless I have a craving for a soda pop. My recommendation is to avoid refined sugars when possible. The natural, non-processed sugars taste better and at the end of the day are probably better for you.

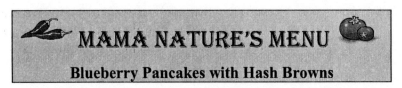

MAMA NATURE'S MENU

Blueberry Pancakes with Hash Browns

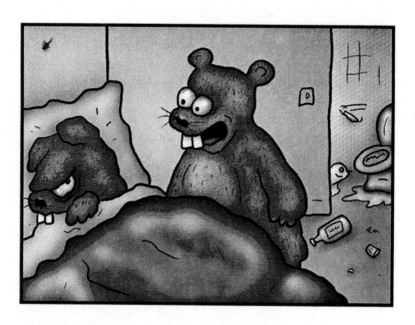

"Well, now we know how much tequila a woodchuck can chuck"

Chapter 9

 Do You Still Need To Take Your Flintstone Chewable Vitamins?

The short answer is no, not if you eat a balanced diet. Iron is an important, essential nutrient because it is a central part of hemoglobin which carries oxygen in the blood to the vital organs. Without sufficient iron in the body, one can get "iron-deficiency anemia". The most common causes are poor diet or blood loss. The most common treatment is simple; increase your iron intake. Iron deficiency is not a problem for a balanced vegan diet. Vegans do not have a higher incidence of iron deficiency than do non-vegans.

Beans and leafy green vegetables are excellent plant sources of iron. Iron absorption is increased by eating foods containing vitamin C, whereas iron absorption is decreased by high levels of caffeine and calcium intake. Many vegetables, such as broccoli and bok choy contain both iron and vitamin C.

According to the USDA, the recommended daily allowances for iron is approximately 10 mg per day for adult men and post-menopausal women and 18 mg per day for pre-menopausal women. The table on the following page shows the iron content of some plant and animal food sources.

Table 7: Selected Food Sources of Iron

Food Item	Serving Size	Iron (mg)
Almonds	¼ cup	1.3
Beef, sirloin	3 oz.	2.0
Broccoli	1 cup	1.1
Clams	3 oz.	23.8
Chicken	½ breast	0.9
Chickpeas	1 cup	4.7
Duck	3 oz.	2.3
Kidney beans	1 cup	5.2
Lentils	1 cup	6.6
Liver	3 oz.	5.2 – 9.9
Molasses	1 tbsp	3.5
Pork chop	3 oz.	0.7
Quinoa	1 cup	6.3
Raisins	½ cup	2.5
Salmon	3 oz.	0.7
Sardines	3 oz.	2.5
Spinach	1 cup	6.4
Tuna	3 oz.	0.8
Capn Crunch®	¾ cup	5.2
Dairy products	n/a	0.0

There has been some research showing that vegetarians have lower levels of iron than non-vegetarians, but not dangerously low levels. Although vegetarians tend to have lower iron stores, they do not have a greater incidence of iron deficiency anemia.

The only research that I came across that was performed solely on vegans was a study performed in Sweden on adolescents. The study found that there was no significant difference in the prevalence of low iron status among vegans and non-vegans.

IRONic Conclusion:

The majority of the research studies that have been performed compare vegetarians (not vegans) to non-vegetarians. One of the reasons that some vegetarians may have lower iron stores is due to their dairy consumption, since dairy contains negligible amounts of iron, and calcium intake has a negative effect on iron retention. Since vegans do not consume dairy, you would expect their iron stores to be satisfactory, which is what the Swedish research concluded. All in all, it is very easy to obtain enough iron from a vegan diet.

Vitamin B12: The curse of the vegan?

Vitamin B12 is a necessary ingredient for the formation of red blood cells, the manufacture of DNA, the proper function of the nervous system, and memory health. Since it is not supplied by plant foods, it is one of the usual "proving points" for non-vegetarians that being a vegetarian is not natural and unhealthy. However, the source of B12 is neither plants nor animals, it is bacteria. Animal foods contain B12 because animals eat foods that are contaminated with bacteria or the bacteria is in the animal's intestine.

Inadequate blood levels of B12 can cause pernicious anemia and nervous system damage. However, low intakes of B12 do not necessarily lead to low supplies in the body. One study indicated that vitamin B12 intake was significantly lower in vegetarians than non-vegetarians, but both groups had similar vitamin B12 levels in their blood. The explanation is that B12 is mainly stored in the liver where a majority of it is reabsorbed by the body instead of excreted. This is the probable reason that it can take over 20 years for deficiencies to develop from inadequate intake.

Vitamin B12 is required in very small amounts. The U.S. recommended intake is approximately 2.4 to 2.8 micrograms (mcgs) a day for ordinary adults. Some people have suggested that foods such as spirulina, seaweed, tempeh, and barley grass are acceptable sources of B12, but that has not been proven.

Most people are in agreement that B12 supplements and fortified foods do provide a reliable source.

Full-blown pernicious anemia is not common among vegans, but is often diagnosed in older people who have difficulty absorbing vitamin B12 from food. Everything that I have read from every source indicates that vegans should take B12 supplements. One of the concerns is memory loss, but I just can't remember the last time I took a B12 vitamin. Achieving an adequate B12 intake is not difficult, simply eat fortified foods or take a supplement.

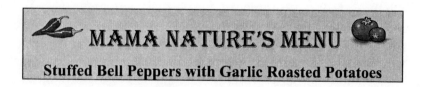

MAMA NATURE'S MENU

Stuffed Bell Peppers with Garlic Roasted Potatoes

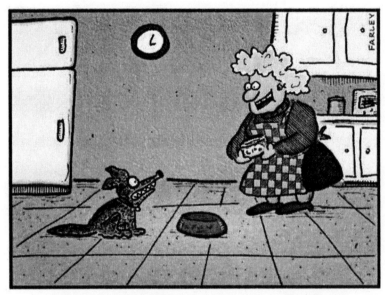

"Oooh- look Muffy! It's sprouts & tofu Alpo!"

Chapter 10

**BUG REPELLENT &
FIELDS OF GENES**
Organic food and
genetically modified food

What is organic food?

"Organic food is produced by farmers who emphasize
the use of renewable resources and the conservation of
soil and water to enhance environmental quality for
future generations. Organic meat, poultry, eggs, and
dairy products come from animals that are given no
antibiotics or growth hormones. Organic food is
produced without using most conventional pesticides;
fertilizers made with synthetic ingredients or sewage
sludge; bioengineering; or ionizing radiation. Before a
product can be labeled as "organic", a Government-
approved certifier inspects the farm where the food is
grown to make sure the farmer is following all the
rules necessary to meet USDA organic standards.
Companies that handle or process organic food before
it gets to your local supermarket or restaurant must be
certified, too."

Is organic food better for you? It appears that this is another one
of those cases where time will tell. Does organic produce taste
better? I think so, but decide for your self.

PRO ORGANIC RESEARCH:

Pesticide Action Network UK: Sixty-five percent of pesticides found as residues in food have been designated by international authorities as having harmful effects on health. Furthermore, toddlers and infants are at risk from residues of toxic pesticides.

Consumer's Union: Pesticide residues are high on some domestic and imported produce, especially for a young child— even one serving of some fruits and vegetables can exceed safe daily limits.

Institute of Food Science & Technology: Organically produced food is more likely to contain lower levels of residues of agricultural chemicals than its non-organic counterparts.

Various Studies: There are significantly more of several nutrients in organic crops. These include: 27% more vitamin C, 21% more iron, 29% more magnesium, and 13% more phosphorus. In addition, organic products contain 15% less nitrates than their conventional counterparts.

American Journal of Agricultural and Food Chemistry: Organic produce contains up to 60 percent more flavonoids, which are cancer-fighting "phytochemicals" and antioxidants.

ANTI ORGANIC OR NEUTRAL RESEARCH

Hudson Institute: Some organic farmers spray their crops with "natural" pesticides, such as pyrethrum, which the EPA has designated as a possible carcinogen.

National Center for Public Policy Research: Some research has suggested that organic farming is only about half as productive as conventional farming, is inadequate in controlling soil erosion, and may have high levels of E-coli bacteria.

United States Department of Agriculture: The USDA makes no claims that organically produced food is safer or more nutritious than conventionally processed food.

Is eating organic food actually better for you? Spraying food with chemicals and injecting animals with needles is a relatively new practice, so it's too early to tell. The evidence is still not clear and you never really know who you can trust, but the thought of someone spraying chemicals on my strawberries makes me a little sick to my stomach. Therefore, I always opt for the organic option when available. Lastly, in my opinion, organic produce actually tastes better. Do your own taste test and decide for yourself.

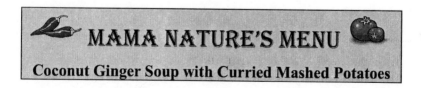

MAMA NATURE'S MENU
Coconut Ginger Soup with Curried Mashed Potatoes

Genetically Modified Foods

Combining genes from different organisms is known as recombinant DNA technology, and the resulting organism is said to be "genetically modified (GM)," "genetically engineered," or "transgenic." In 2003, about 167 million acres grown by 7 million farmers in 18 countries were planted with transgenic crops, mainly insecticide-resistant soybeans, corn, cotton, and canola.

The proposed benefits of GM foods are to reduce maturation time, increase yields, and improve resistance to disease and pests. In other words, increase profits for the producer. The controversies surrounding this technology include the unknown potential human health impact, the unknown effects on biodiversity, and the potential for domination of world food production by a few companies.

The best study that I have found by an independent, reputable organization was performed in March 2004 by the British Medical Association. They found that the potential for GM foods to cause harm is small, however, safety concerns cannot be dismissed completely on the basis of information currently available. In other words, it's too early too tell. We haven't grown any extra limbs as of 2004.

In my opinion, their statement makes sense. It probably does not pose a health risk, but why chance it? We can grow non-modified crops without the risk. My main concern is that many governments, including the U.S, do not require the producer to label food that is genetically modified. Consumers should be able to decide for themselves. Producers have to label everything else, this is equally important.

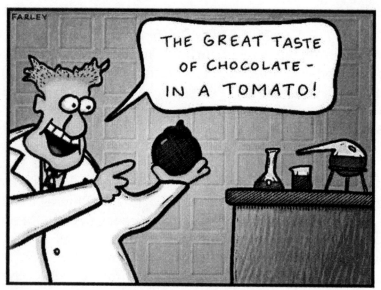

What we have to look forward to from genetic engineering

Chapter 11

FRUIT LOOPS® DON'T GROW ON TREES:
Processed Foods and
Food Additives

Read the ingredients on some of the boxes and cans of food that you have at home. What are all those long names? It doesn't sound like food. Processed foods usually contain chemicals for coloring, flavoring and preserving what was at one time food. You probably suspect that Twinkies® contain some chemicals; how else can they stay fresh for so long?

For your reading enjoyment, here are the ingredients of the beloved Twinkie® (I have **bold-faced** the animal ingredients):

Enriched Wheat Flour - enriched with ferrous sulphate (iron), B vitamins (niacin, thiamine mononitrate [B1], ribofavin [B12] and folic acid), sugar , corn syrup, water, high fructose corn syrup, vegetable and/or **animal shortening** - containing one or more of partially hydrogenated soybean, cottonseed or canola oil, and **beef fat**), dextrose, **whole eggs**, modified corn starch, cellulose gum, **dairy whey**, leavenings (sodium acid pyrophosphate, baking soda, monocalcium phosphate), salt, cornstarch, corn flour, corn syrup solids, **mono and diglycerides**, soy lecithin, polysorbate 60, dextrin, **calcium caseinate**, sodium stearol lactylate, wheat gluten, calcium sulphate, natural and artificial flavors, caramel color, sorbic acid (to retain freshness), color added (yellow 5&6, red 40).

The FDA maintains a list of over 3,000 ingredients added to food. The types of ingredients are preservatives, sweeteners, color additives, flavors, fat replacers, emulsifiers, stabilizers, thickeners, binders, texturizers, leavening agents, anti-caking agents, humectants, yeast nutrients, dough strengtheners and conditioners, firming agents, enzyme preparations, and gases.

Here are some interesting quotes from the FDA:

- Certified colors are synthetically produced and used widely because they impart an intense, uniform color, are less expensive, and blend more easily to create a variety of hues. There are nine certified color additives approved for use in the United States.
- Colors that are exempt from certification include pigments derived from natural sources such as vegetables, minerals or animals. Nature derived color additives are typically more expensive than certified colors and may add unintended flavors to foods.
- Vitamin C or ascorbic acid may be derived from an orange or produced in a laboratory.
- When evaluating the safety of a substance and whether it should be approved, FDA considers: 1) the composition and properties of the substance, 2) the amount that would typically be consumed, 3) immediate and long-term health effects, and 4) various safety factors. The evaluation determines an appropriate level of use that includes a built-in safety margin - a factor that allows for uncertainty about the levels of consumption that are expected to be harmless. In other words, the levels of use that gain approval are much lower than what would be expected to have any adverse effect.
- Because of inherent limitations of science, FDA can never be *absolutely* certain of the absence of any risk from the use of any substance. Therefore, FDA must determine - based on the best science available - if there is a *reasonable certainty of no harm* to consumers when an additive is used as proposed.
- Under the 1958 Food Additives Amendment, two groups of ingredients were exempted from the regulation process. GROUP I - Prior-sanctioned substances - are substances that FDA or USDA had determined safe for use in food prior to the 1958 amendment. Examples are sodium nitrite and potassium nitrite used to preserve luncheon meats. GROUP II - GRAS (generally recognized as safe) ingredients - are those that are generally recognized by experts as safe, based on their extensive history of use in food before 1958 or based on published scientific evidence. Among the several hundred GRAS substances are salt, sugar, spices, vitamins and monosodium glutamate.
- As scientists learn more about the action of certain chemicals in our bodies, FDA uses the new data to reevaluate the permitted use of preservatives. Two examples are the commonly used preservatives BHA and sulfites.

Here are some GRAS ingredients in a Burger King® strawberry milkshake:

> Amyl acetate, amyl butyrate, amyl valerate, anethol, anisyl formate, benzyl acetate, benzyl isobutyrate, butyric acid, cinnamyl isobutyrate, cinnamyl valerate, cognac essential oil, diacetyl, dipropyl ketone, ethyl butyrate, ethyl cinnamate, ethyl heptanoate, ethyl lactate, ethyl methylphenylglycidate, ethyl Nitrate, ethyl propionate, ethyl valerbate, heliotropin, hydroxyphrenyl-2butanone (10% solution in alcohol), a-ionone, isobutyl anthranilate, isobutyl butrate, lemon essential oil, maltol, 4-methylacetophenone, methyl anthranilate, methyl benzoate, methyl cinnamate, methyl heptine carbonate, methyl naphthyl ketone, methyl salicylate, mint essential oil, neroli essential oil, nerolin, neryl isobutyrate, orris butter, phenethyl alcohol, rose, rum ether, g-undecalactone, vanillin, and solvent.

After many years of use, the FDA found food additives that posed health risks and subsequently banned them from use. These include the following: Butter yellow, Green 1, Green 2, Orange 1, Orange 2, Orange B, Red 1, Red 2, Red 4, Red 32, Sudan 1, Violet 1, Yellow 1, Yellow 2, Yellow 3, Yellow 4, cinnamyl anthranilate, cobalt salts, coumarin, cyclamate, diethyl pyrocarbonate, dulcin, ethylene glycol, monochloroacetic acid, nordihydroguaiaretic acid, oil of calamus, polyoxyethylene-8-stearate, safrole, and thiourea.

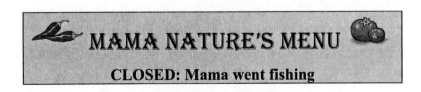

MAMA NATURE'S MENU
CLOSED: Mama went fishing

What are hydrogenated oils and are they bad?

Place a stick of margarine on your open window sill. Return in two years. You will find it in very much the same shape as you left it. Mold won't grow on it and ants won't eat it. What is the reason? Ants and bacteria don't think that hydrogenated oil is food—maybe they're right. Hydrogenation is a process of changing vegetable oil into a more solid form in order to extend the shelf life of various foods. Unfortunately, this process produces trans fatty acids which are found in all hydrogenated or partially hydrogenated vegetable oils, including margarine and shortening. There is a large amount of scientific evidence that says that trans fats are directly linked to an increase in the development of diabetes, cancer, and heart disease.

After closely scrutinizing data from scientific studies and reviews, many European countries have either banned hydrogenated and partially hydrogenated oils altogether or have instituted future dates for elimination of their use in foods.

Many fast foods contain high levels of trans fatty acids. Currently, there are no labeling regulations for fast food, and it can even be advertised as cholesterol-free and cooked in vegetable oil.

Processed Foods That Usually Contain Hydrogenated Oils

Cakes, cookies, muffins and donuts
Crackers
Frozen entrees and meals
Frozen bakery products
French fries
Whipped toppings
Margarines and shortenings
Noodle soup cups
Corn chips and potato chips
Bread, not fresh baked

Are fat substitutes safe?

According to the FDA, fat substitutes are considered safe for limited use, but their long-term benefits and safety are not known.

One popular fat substitute is *Simplesse*, which is made from egg whites and milk proteins. It is created through a process called "microparticulation", in which the protein is shaped into microscopic round particles that roll easily over one another. The end result is a chemical that fools your tongue into thinking that you are eating a creamy fat. Because its components have long been used as foods, the FDA affirmed *Simplesse* as "generally recognized as safe" for use as a thickener or texturizer in frozen dessert products. Safety studies were not required.

Another FDA-approved fat substitute is *Olestra*. This man-made fat substitute provides no calories or fat because your body cannot digest it. It passes directly through your digestive tract and is not absorbed. Health professionals are unsure of the effect of *Olestra* on the gastrointestinal system and of the effect on the absorption of other nutrients.

It is too early to tell if there are any health benefits and/or health risks from using products with fat substitutes. In my opinion, there is nothing wrong with fat as long as it comes from the right sources. Your body needs fat, what it doesn't need is saturated fat loaded with cholesterol.

Monosodium glutamate (MSG)

MSG is a flavor enhancer produced through the fermentation of corn, sugar beets or sugar cane. MSG elicits a unique taste that is known as "umami" in Japan, and often described by Americans as a savory, broth-like or meaty flavor. In the United

States, MSG has been included in the FDAs list of substances known as generally recognized as safe since 1959.

The FDA claims that MSG is safe when it is consumed at "usual" levels by the general population. However, the FDA has identified some short-term adverse reactions to MSG. Some people may have a reaction after eating large doses of MSG, particularly on an empty stomach. A typical serving of glutamate-treated food contains less than 0.5 grams of MSG, whereas a large dose would be 3 grams or more. The FDA also recommends that people with asthma stay away from MSG.

Due to bad publicity, food manufacturers have found ways to hide MSG. They list the ingredients that contain MSG but not the MSG itself. For example, broth, which may contain MSG can be listed as an ingredient on a label, but the ingredients in the broth are not required to be listed.

TABLE 8: Food Additives and MSG

Food Additives That Always Contain MSG	Food Additives That Frequently Contain MSG
Hydrolyzed Vegetable Protein	Malt Extract
Hydrolyzed Protein	Malt Flavoring
Plant Protein Extract	Bouillon
Sodium Caseinate	Broth
Calcium Caseinate	Stock
Yeast Extract	Flavoring
Textured Protein	Natural Flavors/Flavoring
Autolyzed Yeast	Seasoning
Hydrolyzed Oat Flour	Spices

MSG is vegan, but is it safe or not? At low levels of consumption, it appears to be safe, but if you have asthma it is probably best to stay away from it. Why are we adding flavor enhancers to our food anyway? There's plenty of food out there that tastes good on its own without making it taste like something else. Enough with the fake food already.

Conclusion:

Processing takes a lot of the nutrients and enzymes out of foods. There is nothing wrong with eating food as it occurs in nature. Don't let the food industry fool you into thinking it can manufacture healthy foods. That is nature's job. The less food is processed and altered, the easier your body can process it and the better it is for your health. Whenever you take a food from nature and change its composition or strip nutrients from it, you will always have less nutritional benefits. Mother Nature knows best.

DID YOU KNOW?

Many brands of canned meats have no expiration date.

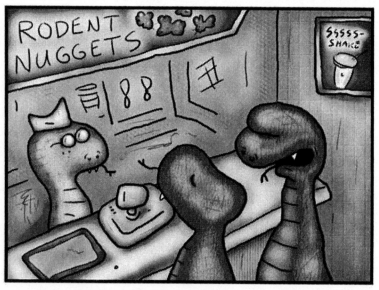

"You don't really know what's in those things."

Chapter 12

"30 DAYS TO LEAVE YOUR BLUBBER"™

> "Thou shouldst eat to live; not live to eat"
> - *Socrates* (469 BC – 399 BC)
>
> "As a child my mother's menu had two choices: take it or leave it."
> - *Unknown*

The *30 Days to Leave Your Blubber*™ program is a gradual process of cutting meat, poultry, fish and dairy out of your diet over approximately 30 days. The first week, we cut it out of the morning meal. The second week, we do the same to lunch. In week 3, we tackle dinner. In the final week, we put the finishing touches on the daily routine. The 30 days is not "set in stone", it is a guideline—this is your program, you set the pace.

Treat the 30 days as a golden opportunity to evaluate and re-evaluate the way you currently eat. Experiment and find foods that you like, and the foods that nourish and treat your body right.

WATCH YOUR BODY CHANGE

You may drop a few waist sizes. Don't be alarmed. Your skin may become clearer. Don't be alarmed. Your cholesterol level may drop dramatically. Don't be alarmed. You may want to go hug a tree and pet a baby chick. Be alarmed.

You will lose weight. How much is hard to say; everyone is different. The point of this program is not to count the pounds and inches that go away, but to get your body into its intended, natural, healthy state. Losing unnecessary fat is simply a byproduct of eating healthy. Eating healthy is not about counting calories, assigning points to tomatoes, or doing any other crazy schemes to lose weight. It is about eating whatever you want, when you want. You are cleaning your body. Your body is going to change for the better.

LISTEN TO YOUR BODY

Your body will tell you what it needs, as well as what it does not need. Your body is the boss—your mind just works there full time. If you give your body what it needs, when it needs it, it will function naturally. If you ignore your body, it will nag and complain and eventually break down.

Listening to your body means paying attention to what you eat and how it affects you. If you eat a particular food item and it makes you feel bloated and lethargic, cut it out of your regular diet. Stay away from foods that make you walk like a penguin. If you eat a food item and you have trouble taking out the trash the next day (i.e. you are constipated), cut back on it. Give your body clean-burning fuel that keeps it functioning naturally.

Trust the wisdom of your body and eating will become a natural function, just like sleeping. When you are tired, you sleep. When you are hungry, you eat. When you are not hungry, don't eat. You will find your way to better health and vitality when you listen to your body.

Eating the vegan way is not a form of punishment or abstinence from enjoying food. Eat whatever you want, when you want it. If you have a taste for something sweet, eat something sweet. If you have a taste for something crunchy and salty, get after it. If you have a taste for a big lobster tail smothered in butter, go to your room and lock the door.

EAT LESS PROCESSED FOODS

Remember that food is fuel—the cleaner the fuel, the better your body will function. As a general rule, the more processed food is, the further it has changed from its original, natural state, and the harder it is for your body to process and digest it. Artificial flavorings, colorings and preservatives are not food, they are chemicals. Try to limit your intake of processed foods and eat what Mother Nature provides, not a scientist in a laboratory.

DRINK WATER

Water is the most necessary ingredient in your body. It carries nutrients to your cells and waste away from your cells. It is the main ingredient in blood and it keeps your bones and joints lubricated. Water keeps the digestive system working properly, and is the key ingredient in moving food through your body and out the back door. Keeping food moving along the digestive system is vital to your health. So drink lots of water all day long.

In general, women should consume approximately nine 8-oz. glasses of water each day and men should consume roughly twelve 8-oz. glasses of water each day. The more water that you drink, the more your body will cleanse, the less hungry you will be, and the more your body will be in balance.

ATTITUDE

Freedom is having the ability to do what you want to do when you want to do it. Attitude is having the inner strength to exercise that freedom. Eating is a conscious activity. Don't do it unconsciously.

You possess the capacity to say yes as well as the capacity to say no. Yes is always easier when it comes to eating. Attitude is about perfecting your level of self-control to the point where your mind rules both your body and spirit. Attitude is having the strength to say "no way Jose".

Discipline is simply looking straight ahead

OK, but what am I going to EAT?

You may not realize this yet, but you probably already eat some meals that are vegan. More importantly, you can probably make some modifications to meals that you already eat. It may be as simple as leaving off the cheese. For example, pasta with marinara sauce is vegan if you leave off the Parmesan cheese, and pizza is delicious without the cheese.

It is not difficult or boring to be vegan. There are hundreds of vegan soup and chili variations, hundreds of salad variations, hundreds of sandwich options, etc. You can make or eat meals that are basic or gourmet, it's up to you. You can still go out to eat at restaurants. Your lifestyle does not have to change, but being a vegan will change your life.

I will give you some additional guidance for meals later on in this chapter. For now, just keep in mind that there is more to it than tofu and sprouts. In the end, however, it will be your responsibility to find the foods that you like and dislike—and you will have fun finding those foods.

Snacks and Snacking

If you are hungry, eat. If you are used to snacking throughout the day, feel free to continue to do so. You can eat potato chips, tortilla chips, pretzels, microwave popcorn, trail mix, wasabi peas, rice cakes, energy bars and much more. You can also snack on nuts, vegetables and dried fruit such as figs and raisins. A mid-afternoon smoothie also makes a great snack. Eventually, try to substitute fruits and vegetables for chips and pretzels.

How and When to Start

You have to prepare mentally and refrigeratingly for this journey (i.e. you have to stock your refrigerator). I recommend shopping at a new grocery store, for the simple reason of breaking the old habit of going to the dairy section or the meat counter. It is not a requirement to shop at a "healthy grocery store" such as Whole Foods™ or Wild Oats™, although it would probably help in the beginning. These health food stores have a vast array of options.

Start on a Monday, everyone starts stuff on Mondays, so why be different? You're not going to start on a Wednesday; nobody does that. How about starting this coming Monday?

On Sunday night, try this. Call your favorite pizza parlor and order a cheeseless pizza. I do it all the time, they may laugh, but who cares—they'll deliver it. Put any veggies on the pizza that you want—my mainstay is mushroom, onion, tomato and hot giardiniera.

Eat and enjoy the pizza, and mentally prepare for your journey. If you are ordering with a friend, most pizza places can make half the pizza with cheese and the other half without. I always get a big laugh, but they do it anyway. "You wanta pizza witha halfa cheese? Whatta you a crazy vegan?"

Table 9: Some recommended staples for your kitchen:

Bulk Food Section	Frozen Food Section
Brown rice	Veggie burgers & dogs
Quinoa- see below	Vegan sausage
Lentils	Frozen meals
Raisins, dates, and figs	Bag of spinach and corn
Nutritional yeast- see below	Non-dairy ice cream
Granola	Frozen fruit bars

Grocery Section	Refrigerated Section
Bragg™ Liquid Aminos	Hommus
Soy sauce or tamari	Tempeh- see below
Canned beans	Seitan- see below
Canned soups	Miso- see below
Bread	Fruit juices
Bagels	Ready-made burritos
Crackers	Soy yogurt
Tortilla chips	Salsa
Popcorn	Guacamole
Rice cakes	
Snack bars	**Produce Section**
Pasta	Fruit and vegetables
Tomato sauce	Baby carrots for snacks
Soy milk or rice milk	Collard greens
Peanut butter	Bok choy
Almond butter	Potatoes
Maple syrup	Fresh herbs and spices
Olive & canola oil	Brussel sprouts
Unbleached flour	-give the lil' guy a chance

Rice: I recommend short grain brown rice. White rice is just naked brown rice (the bran portion and fiber removed). If you eat brown rice, you can throw away your Metamucil and fiber pills. For cooking rice, see Appendix 1.

Quinoa: Quinoa, pronounced (keen-wah), originated in the Andes mountains of South America and was a staple of the Incan civilization. Quinoa contains more protein than any other grain and can be substituted for rice in any dish. It tastes really good and is quick and easy to prepare, see Appendix 1.

Nutritional yeast: Nutritional yeast is a complete protein and contains many of the B-vitamins, including B12. It has a unique flavor, similar to Parmesan cheese. It is a great "sprinkle-on" condiment for many dishes, such as pizza and stir fries.

Bragg™ Liquid Aminos: This stuff rocks. It is a liquid protein concentrate, similar to a soy sauce or tamari. However, it is not fermented, heated and is gluten free. It has a very unique flavor and is great on everything. Add this to popcorn with some nutritional yeast—trust me, it may not sound good, but you will never miss buttered popcorn.

Soy milk, almond milk, rice milk: Don't be afraid of this stuff—food producers have made it very tasty. Most of the brands fortify the milk with calcium, vitamin D, and B12. They also have various flavors including vanilla, chocolate and carob. Use on cereals, in soups, sauces, and baked goods.

Nut butters: Nut butters are packed with protein. There are many varieties and brands of nut butters out there. Choose one that has no additives at all—only nuts. If you have never tasted almond butter, do yourself a huge favor and get a small jar. If you like peanut butter, you will love almond butter. I put it in smoothies or eat it straight out of the jar. Try it on toast and put a little sweetener on top, such as maple syrup and raisins.

Veggie burgers & dogs: There are many options to choose from. Experiment until you find the ones that you like the best. The majority of them tend to be very processed—so don't make veggie burgers and hot dogs an everyday meal, rather a special treat, or when you have time constraints. If you are going to eat a lot of them, I recommend eating a salad or steamed vegetables as a side dish.

Vegan sausage: Again, there are many options to choose from. They come in all shapes and sizes—links, patties, strips, and crumbled. My favorite is Lightlife GimmeLean® Sausage.

Tempeh: Tempeh is made from fermented soybeans. Tempeh has many nutrients and is much more flavorful and has a better texture than tofu. It is great in stir fries and if shredded can easily take the place of ground beef. See my recipe for tempeh tacos in Appendix 1.

Seitan: Seitan is a meat alternative. It was invented for the sole reason to replace meat—and it does a great job. It works well in veggie fajitas, and deli-style sandwiches. It is essentially wheat gluten, processed and spiced up. It's a good option if you have a craving for "meat" during the beginning of the program.

TVP (texturized vegetable protein): TVP is another meat alternative. It is made from soy flour which has been cooked, extruded and dried. It is high in nutrients and has the consistency of ground meat. This is processed food made to think you are eating meat.

Soy cheese: There are many flavors and brands of soy cheese. Some are very good, while some taste like rubber. Experiment until you find the brands that you like. You'll have to read the labels, since some soy cheeses contain caseinate which is derived from milk.

Miso: Miso is made from fermented soy beans. There are many different types of miso that vary in flavor. In Japan, different types of miso are prepared and evaluated much the way we judge fine wines. Use miso to flavor soups, sauces, dressings and marinades. One-quarter cup in a quart of water makes a savory soup stock.

Collard greens: This green vegetable looks like it's from the Fred Flintstone era. Trust me on this one, try it. Chop them up anyway that looks good to you and steam with some water and Braggs™, and add some garlic powder. Collard greens also are a great addition to any veggie stir fry. They have a great flavor and are loaded with nutrients.

"If we don't change our direction, we're likely to end up where we are headed."
-Chinese Proverb

WARNING:
POSSIBLE GAS
ATTACK

Anytime that your diet changes, your body may have a reaction. If you have not eaten a lot of raw salads and veggies throughout your life, it may take your body a few days to adjust. Your body will eventually get accustomed to your new way of eating, just like it did before. Be patient with nature. If you have the farts for a few days, big deal. Blame the dog.

Table 10: Names for farts in different languages:

Dej – Danish	Doofu – Ethiopian
Fang Pi – Chinese	Fing – Hungarian
Fuss – Lebanese	Furz – German
Paad – Hindi	Gooz – Persian
Trump – English	Puk – Russian
Crepidus – Latin	Bram – Welsh
1 Cheek Sneak – American	General Colon Bowel - American

EATING AT
RESTAURANTS

> "The problem with eating Italian food is that a week later, you're hungry again"
> -*Unknown*

Fact: Restaurants are a "for profit" business

Fact: Profits ↑ as Costs ↓

Fact: $E = mc^2$

It's all relative, but for most restaurants, the object is to charge as much as they can and pay as little as possible for the ingredients, while making the food taste great so you come back for more. Usually this implies that the ingredients are inferior to what you can obtain on your own. Ingredients are usually processed to increase shelf lives, have additives to make them look appealing, and have a high fat content to make it taste yummy. National restaurant chains have boards of directors and shareholders who demand profits, so be skeptical of the quality of the food.

Don't get me wrong, I enjoy going out to eat. I love to cook, but I'm not doing dishes every night! All restaurants are not created equal, many restaurants serve quality food. You do not have to avoid going out to eat, just be prepared to ask questions. As a consumer you have a right to know what you are eating, so don't feel bad about asking. Some foods have "hidden" animal ingredients that you might want to avoid, for example, some pasta sauces are made with chicken stock and some salad dressings contain mayonnaise.

Here is an example of how I got bamboozled:

> I am at an Italian restaurant, craving pasta with a spicy tomato sauce. The only dish available has ground sausage in it. I kindly ask the waiter to ask the chef if he can make the dish without the sausage. The waiter returns and says, "the chef says of course, no problem". I drink a glass of wine, get involved in conversation, eat half of my meal, and then stop abruptly. Something doesn't exactly taste right. I poke around in my plate and sure enough there are pieces of sausage in the food. I ask the waiter to please ask the chef what happened. The chef comes out and says "I tried my best to pick the sausage out of the sauce".

Was I angry? Yes, a little. Did it kill me? No. Did I finish the bottle of wine? Probably, but I don't remember. The moral of the story is that you have to be careful at restaurants and not be afraid to ask lots of repeated questions. Another short anecdote comes from 1990 in Hot Springs, Arkansas.

> I am at another Italian restaurant. I open the menu, not expecting to find anything to eat. But lo and behold, there is a vegetarian section of the menu. Upon further review, it only contained one menu item- "Chicken Primavera".

Chicken is poultry, it's not beef—so they thought it was vegetarian! Fortunately, restaurants have come a long way since then. In addition to Italian restaurants, you can usually find options at Chinese, Indian and Thai restaurants. These types of restaurants offer a variety of vegan dishes. However, make sure there are no fish sauces in the dishes, especially the soups.

Mexican restaurants always have options and are usually accommodating. Chips, salsa, guacamole and veggie burritos are regular menu items. Most Mexican restaurants do not use lard in their refried beans anymore, but it never hurts to ask.

Another great option is sushi. If you have never tried sushi, I recommend checking it out. You can create your own sushi rolls using ingredients such as avocado, cucumber, spinach, asparagus, mushrooms, carrots and jalapenos. You can also order gomai, which is steamed spinach with sesame sauce, and edamame, which are cooked soybeans—they are really good.

Other tips for ordering at restaurants:

1. **Pasta:** Make sure it is dried pasta not egg pasta, usually the angel hair is a safe bet.

2. **Sauces:** Ask how the sauce is prepared, do they use oil, butter or chicken stock?

3. **Fried food:** Many restaurants fry all their food in the same fryer. So, the french fries are probably fried in the same oil as the chicken wings.

4. **Veggie Burgers:** Many veggie burgers are made with cheese, so it doesn't hurt to ask.

5. **Salad Dressings:** If it's white, it usually contains dairy. The safest way to go is with oil and vinegar.

6. **No Cheese/No Butter:** Always assume they are going to slap butter on baked potatoes and toast, and cheese on everything, even if it's not listed on the menu.

Do not be afraid of going out to eat, your social life does not have to change. It may take some time to figure out where you can go and how to order. It is always a good idea to call the restaurant ahead of time and see what options are on the menu.

WEEK 1:
GIVE BREAKFAST
A FACELIFT

> "Never eat more than you can lift."
> - *Miss Piggy*

The morning meal is the most important part of the program. Morning is the time of day where your body wants to take out the garbage from the day before, so let it. When you wake up in the morning, your body is cleansing. Try not to load it up with too much stuff, allow it to do its work efficiently. You brush your teeth everyday so that you have healthy teeth; cleanse your body every morning so that you have a healthy system.

The best thing to eat in the morning is fresh fruit and juices. Fruit requires a small amount of energy to digest, therefore, allowing your body to focus its energy on other things, such as reading the morning newspaper. Fruit also assists your body's natural effort to cleanse in the morning. The cleaner the fuel, the cleaner your body—the healthier you will feel. You can eat fruit all morning long.

You do not have to give up your morning coffee, it is not going to hurt you. However, dunking six jelly donuts in it will. Remember, however, that too much caffeine will start to leach calcium from your bones. One to three cups of coffee a day is usually fine, but when you start to drink more, you are entering the risky zone.

If you want to eat more than fruit at first, then ask yourself what do you typically eat in the morning? If it's a cup of coffee with a bagel or muffin, make or buy some. If it's a bowl of cereal, eat a bowl of cereal. If you like oatmeal, eat oatmeal—try it with a splash of maple syrup. If it's the weekend, and you normally make pancakes and sausage—do it, there are great vegan sausages available. See Appendix 1 for recipes for muffins and pancakes.

If you need some help getting started, here are some simple suggestions for breakfast.

THE QUICK & EASY

FRUITS & JUICES: Any fruit is a good fruit: oranges, grapefruits, melons, bananas, etc. Eat fruit and drink juice all morning.

SMOOTHIES: If you have a blender, you're in business. You can make anything into a smoothie. Start with bananas and ice and add fruit, such as strawberries, raspberries, peaches, and apples. For a twist, add cocoa, cinnamon, coconut, or a shot of espresso. If you need a protein boost, add some almond or peanut butter. If you prefer your smoothies sweet, add a shot of maple syrup.

CEREALS & GRANOLA: There are many flavors and brands of granola and breakfast cereals. Many are vegan. In fact, Cap'n Crunch® is vegan, but loaded with refined sugar and additives. If you like hot cereal, have some oatmeal.

BAGELS, TOAST & ENGLISH MUFFINS: Most are vegan. However, if a bagel has a shiny coat, that generally means it has been dipped in an egg wash. Instead of butter and cream cheese, try soy margarine or vegan cream cheeses.

BREAKFAST SANDWICHES: Try making a vegan vegmuffin. Use a toasted bagel or English muffin. Add soy cheese and a vegan sausage patty.

HASH BROWNS: There are many variations of hash browns. They are not difficult to make at home. See Appendix 1 for recipe.

PANCAKES: Vegan pancakes are easy to prepare. You can make apple pancakes, blueberry pancakes, banana pancakes, and chocolate chip pancakes, just to name a few. See Appendix 1 for recipe.

FRENCH TOAST: Guess what? This is easy to make as well. See Appendix 1 for recipe.

BLUEBERRY MUFFINS: There are countless varieties of muffins. You can make a big batch and freeze them. See Appendix 1 for recipe.

GREASY SPOON BREAKFAST: We all like the occasional belly-filling, greasy breakfast. For the ultimate greasy spoon breakfast, see the recipe for "Hangover Helper" in Appendix 1.

Restaurants for breakfast

Unless you eat at a vegetarian restaurant, your breakfast options may be limited, but not hopeless. You can always find oatmeal and fruit and some restaurants offer soy milk with their breakfast cereals. You can also usually order hash browns and toast, as most restaurants cook their hash browns in oil.

The rest of the day, eat as you normally would. If you want to cut back on your meat and dairy intake the rest of the day, have at it. Do not be afraid to experiment, you will find new foods that you like to eat. Remember to drink lots of water all day long and keep listening to the boss—your body.

WEEK 2:
WHAT'S FOR
LUNCH

> "Ask not what you can do for your country. Ask what's for lunch."
> *-Orson Welles* (1915-1985)

Ask yourself what you normally eat in the afternoon. If it's yogurt and a candy bar, try soy yogurt and a granola bar—there are some really great flavors available. If you normally eat soup and salad or a sandwich, there are hundreds of options available. If you normally eat a bacon cheeseburger, fries and a milkshake, you have some work to do, but it won't be as difficult as you may think.

The best thing to do for lunch is bring your own. Prepare your own lunch in the morning or bring leftovers or ready-made meals. If "brown-bagging" is not an option, then be prepared to ask questions at restaurants. You will eventually figure out where to go and what to order.

I want to reiterate the importance of discovering new foods to eat. Walk the aisles of a "healthy" grocery store and see what looks appealing. Don't be afraid to try something that you never heard of—it's not going to harm you. Some of it will taste like an old shoe, but you will find many foods that you like. The suggestions that I list in this book are just the beginning; they are the tip of the iceberg lettuce.

If you need some help getting started, here are some simple suggestions for lunch.

THE QUICK & EASY

SANDWICHES: Make a hommus sandwich with any toppings such as tomato, onions and sprouts. Try it on sourdough, a bagel or stuffed into a pita pocket. Try a peanut butter and banana sandwich on cinnamon raisin bread. There are also vegan deli-style meats available.

SOY YOGURT & GRANOLA BAR: There are many varieties of soy yogurts and granola bars. By the way, they are nutritious and delicious.

READY-MADE SOUPS: There are many soups available in a can, or in a bowl. Keep a stockpile at work.

BURRITOS & WRAPS: There are many already-made burritos and veggie wraps available. Pack one of these in your briefcase, purse or backpack.

THE NOT SO QUICK BUT EASY

VEGGIE BURRITOS: Make your own with pinto beans, rice, lettuce, tomato, onion, guacamole and salsa. Most of the time, both corn and flour tortillas are vegan.

GRILLED PORTABELLA SANDWICH: Grill up a portabella mushroom and put it on your favorite bread. Try it on dark rye bread with grilled onions and soy cheese. For a twist, sauté it in Bragg™ and garlic powder.

HOME-MADE SOUPS: Make your own soup, it's as easy as making soup. See Appendix 1 for recipes.

93

Restaurants for lunch

If you live or work in a city, there are probably restaurants that you can go to. Do an internet search for vegan-friendly restaurants in your area. If the only alternatives are chain fast food restaurants, or food courts, SUBWAY® has vegan options. According to their website, the Veggie Delite® is vegan and the wheat bread and deli roll contain honey but no other animal-derived products.

If you want a super healthy jolt of nutritious energy, find a juice bar. You may not like some of the juice combinations at first, so start with plain old carrot juice. Then start experimenting with other veggies. Fruit smoothies are also an option.

~~~~~~~~~~~~~~~

If you do not feel like you are getting enough energy during the day, then increase what you are eating. Try incorporating nut butters into your daily diet. If your body needs protein, give it some. Keep a bag of snacks on hand. Find out what works best for you.

If possible, try to avoid eating a big meal in the afternoon—save it for dinner. Keep the fuel clean and easy to process. If you want to continue to eat fruit (including smoothies) throughout the afternoon, and keep your body on cleanse mode, have at it. The rest of the day, and dinnertime, eat as you normally would. Again, keep in mind that the less your food is processed, the better. Don't forget to drink water all day long.

WEEK 3:
♪ THE NIGHT TIME IS THE RIGHT TIME FOR MAKIN' VEGGIES ♪

"Our bodies are our gardens to which our wills are gardeners"
-*William Shakespeare* (1564-1616)

"I cook with wine. Sometimes I even add it to the food."
-*W.C. Fields* (1880-1946)

Eating is the most important activity of the day, so devote as much time to it as possible. If you normally "veg out" on the couch and watch television, steal a half hour and use it for preparing a meal. You may discover that you enjoy preparing food.

If you do not think that you can cook, think again. Do you know how to barbeque? Then you know how to cook. Can you put rice in a pot, add water, and turn on the stove? Then you can cook. Can you chop up veggies, add spices, and throw them in a pan? Then you can cook. Can you boil water and cook pasta? Then you can cook. Treat cooking as a vacation from the outside world's noise. Turn off the cell phone and make yourself a decent meal—treat yourself right.

You can turn almost any recipe into a gourmet vegan meal. If you have a recipe for ravioli, try stuffing them with sautéed spinach and mushrooms. You can make vegan enchiladas, spinach pie, and minestrone soup. The possibilities are endless, and by the way, are good for you.

There is never enough time in a day, and realistically, you are not going to have time every night to cook, so be prepared. When you make rice, make enough for two nights. Make sure your kitchen is stocked with veggie burgers, bagels, hommus, and canned soups.

If you need some help getting started, here are some simple suggestions for dinner.

THE QUICK & EASY

VEGGIE BURGER & OVEN FRIES: There are many varieties of veggie burgers and many ways to prepare them. If you're in a rush, you can always toss one in the microwave. Try serving a veggie burger on a bagel—it's a good combination.

PASTA PRIMAVERA: Make your favorite pasta and tomato sauce. Chop up some veggies, such as carrots, broccoli, mushrooms and spinach, and add them to the sauce. Voila - pasta primavera.

BEAN & CORN BURRITOS: Open a can of beans and a frozen bag of corn. Put in a pot, and add spices. Warm up corn or flour tortillas. Break out the salsa, guacamole and other condiments. Wrap it, eat it, enjoy it, and sing *"La Cucaracha"*.

PIZZA & SALAD: When in doubt, the yellow pages get brought out. When you have time constraints, you can always order a cheeseless pizza and a salad.

LASAGNA: There are many lasagna variations. I have included a recipe for spinach mushroom lasagna in Appendix 1.

VEGGIE STIR FRY: Experiment with veggies that you have never tried before, such as collard greens, kale and bok choy. Try adding potatoes, including sweet potatoes to your stir fries. Add a can of black beans, red beans or white beans—they come in all colors. Serve over brown rice or quinoa.

BBQ: Good news! You don't have to retire your barbeque. Most barbeque sauces are vegan—you can also make your own. You can make veggie skewers with anything such as mushrooms, onions, peppers, zucchini, and more. You can also grill potatoes and corn on the cob. Try adding tempeh to your veggie skewers—it's good stuff.

Restaurants for dinner

As previously mentioned, there are many possibilities—you just have to be prepared to ask questions. Most of the time, you will find that restaurant staff are accommodating, since this type of diet is becoming more mainstream every day (and they want a decent tip).

You don't have to sacrifice eating out at restaurants. You just have to make a trade-off—trading in the Chicken Parmesan for Pasta Primavera and a healthier body. It's fun to go out to eat—no question. It's even more fun to go out to eat and smile in the mirror everyday. After awhile, you may even discover that "fine dining" happens in your own kitchen.

WEEK 4:
VEGANBURGER
IN PARADISE

"Every man is the builder of a temple called his body."
-*Henry David Thoreau* (1817-1862)

The fourth week is the fine-tuning week. By this time, you will have found some great new foods that you are enjoying. However, it may not be going 100 percent perfect. If you are still putting a little milk or cream in your coffee, it's not the end of the world. However, try to substitute soy milk. If you are still putting Parmesan cheese on your food, try to substitute nutritional yeast or soy cheese. Give this program a solid, focused effort—give it a chance, that way you will know if it is right for you.

If you are having a difficult time, ask yourself why? What are you missing or craving? If you miss cutting into a piece of meat, try grilling a portabella mushroom and throw some A1® sauce on it. If you are craving ice cream, there are many outrageous vegan options. If you are having difficulty finding a variety of foods to eat, walk into a healthy grocery store and see what they offer in the prepared foods section. You can also look in the frozen section to find ready-made meals that you may like. There are also hundreds of free vegan recipes and suggestions on the internet.

It takes time for your body to adjust to change. It is not easy to quit smoking in a day—same with your diet. It gets easier as time goes by—trust me. I ate bacon and eggs for breakfast, chicken for lunch, and beef for dinner for years. Making the transition took time and effort, but in hindsight, it was not that difficult. You will be thankful in the long run.

If you fall off the program, jump back on or start over from week number one. You can also stretch each week into two weeks, or longer. Take your time, set your own pace, nobody is watching. Remember that you are doing something good for your body and yourself. Don't be afraid of change.

 # Rules of the Road for Week 4

Watch your body change.

Trust the wisdom of your body.

Attitude is having the strength to say NO.

Discipline is simply looking straight ahead.

Eat, drink and be merry.

TRAVELLING

It is usually not difficult to find food when you travel. Take some time and plan. Before you depart, do an internet search for vegan-friendly restaurants and health food stores in the area, or grab a yellow pages when you arrive at your destination.

Most major airlines now offer vegan meals—you just have to order it ahead of time. Sometimes it's a peanut butter and jelly sandwich, other times it's a little more interesting. You can always bring your own food, if you can get it through security.

It is also a good idea to learn the words for "no cheese" in the language of the country that you are traveling to.

> Spanish- no queso
> French- aucun fromage
> German- kein kase
> Italian- nessuno formaggio
> Dutch- geen kaas
> Portuguese- nenhum queijo
> Norwegian- ingen ost
> Russian- никакой сыр
> Chinese- 没有奶酪

Es no problema para viajar: It is no problem to travel

Imagine sitting on a beach in Mexico watching the sun go down. It's a pleasant 78.5°F with a slight breeze. Your toes are in the sand. On the table next to you is a plate with fresh guacamole, fresh salsa, fresh tortilla chips and a pineapple with an umbrella sticking out of it… what's the problem?

THE SWEET
TOOTH VEGAN

"Stressed spelled backwards is desserts."
-*Unknown*

"Coffee, chocolate, and men; some things are just better rich."
-*Unknown*

You do not have to give up your sweet tooth. However, you will have to give up the Crème Brule and Baked Alaska. There are many options, here are just a few.

Frozen Desserts: Sorbet (not Sherbet) is usually vegan. There are also many "ice creams" available now that are very good. There are flavors such as chocolate mint, chocolate fudge, french vanilla, praline pecan, and cookies 'n' cream, just to name a few. There are also many flavors of frozen fruit bars. There's even a chocolate covered frozen banana that is awesome. You can also peel some ripe bananas and toss them in your freezer—they make a great snack or frozen dessert.

Candy Bars: There are many candy bars out there as well. Tropical Source® makes chocolate bars with flavors such as hazelnut, rice crisp, toasted almond, mint crunch and raspberry. Yum!

Puddings: You can make or buy vegan chocolate puddings. You can also make banana pudding, rice pudding, and many more flavors. By the way, they taste great.

Muffins, Cookies, Brownies, Pies, and Cakes: You can turn any traditional dessert into a vegan delicacy. How does amaretto peach upside down cake sound? Or chocolate raspberry cake, with macadamia nut frosting? What about pumpkin pie, cherry pecan pie, peanut butter and chocolate cookies, blueberry muffins, and chocolate brownies? The possibilities are endless.

The Best Chocolate Dessert on the Planet: If you are a chocoholic, try making this dessert. You will not believe that it is vegan. Make this for friends and see what happens. See Appendix 1 for recipe.

It will not be difficult to satisfy your sweet tooth.

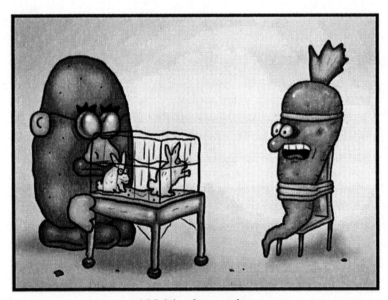

1984 in the garden

Chapter 13

**FINAL THOUGHTS
AND SUGGESTIONS**

The beautiful thing about this diet is that everything you are going to eat is good for you. You don't have to sacrifice your love for eating. Have fun with this experience and try different foods. If you have some difficulty figuring out what to eat, there are many free resources on the web such as recipes and lists of vegan friendly restaurants in your area.

If you don't make it the entire thirty days, hop back on whenever you are ready. Try it again, or incorporate the vegan diet into your life whenever and however you want. You make the rules.

If you decide that this vegan stuff is for the birds, let me make one last suggestion. Continue to eat meat, but cut out dairy and processed foods from your diet. Our bodies are set up to process simple, natural foods, not another animal's milk or food created in a laboratory. I'm not talking about fried meats or scrap meats loaded with fillers (i.e. chicken wings and hotdogs). If you are going to eat meat, eat a lean, clean piece of meat.

The bottom line is to do what you think is best for your body. Find out for yourself. Start today. The better the effort you put forth, the better the results. The vegan diet may not be for you, but then again, it could be the most important thing that you have ever done.

At the time of the first publication of this book, I'm reaching 40 years of age. I have never felt healthier. I may have lost a step on my niece and nephews, and my back may be a bit stiffer in the morning; but deep down, I am the healthiest that I have ever been. Every year that I continue to eat healthy, I feel better. Enjoy life from the healthy side of the fence. Live long enough so you can use up your frequent flyer miles.

> "It's not the years in your life that count. It's the life in your years"
> -*Abraham Lincoln* (1809-1865)

≈≈≈≈≈≈≈≈≈≈≈≈≈≈≈≈≈≈≈≈≈≈≈≈≈≈≈≈≈≈

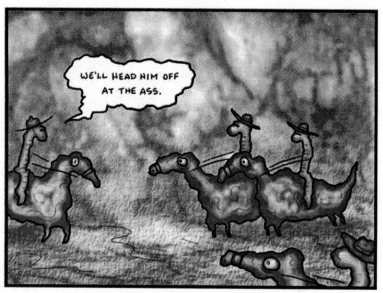

Tapeworm Posse

Appendix 1

MAMA NATURE'S
MENU
(Recipes)

There are volumes of vegan cookbooks. There are also free recipes on the internet. What I have included here are some simple, fun ones. The only recipes that you need to strictly adhere to are the ones for cooking rice and making muffins and pancakes. All the other recipes are just guidelines—modify them as you deem appropriate. The beautiful thing about these recipes is that you cannot screw them up. You may even improve them.

COOKING RICE & QUINOA

Brown Rice: The rice to water ratio is 1 cup of rice to 1 ½ cups of water. If you have an automatic rice cooker, cook until the rice is soft and dry. Otherwise, use a sauce pan, cover and heat until a rapid boil. Lower heat and continue to cook until the rice is soft and dry. Try adding Bragg™ and any spices that you like to the cooked rice.

Quinoa: Use 1 cup of quinoa to 1 ½ cups of water. Bring to a boil, cover and turn off heat. It is ready to eat in 15 minutes. Add your favorite sauces and seasonings.

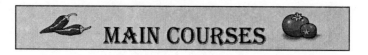

MAIN COURSES

Soup is great food

Making soup from scratch is easy. You can make a fresh soup from scratch in 30 minutes or less once you get good at it. Again, recipes are important if you are baking a cake—we're making soup here, not Quiche Lorraine.

SOUP BASE

Ingredients:
2 garlic cloves or 1 tbsp of garlic powder
1 medium sized yellow onion
2 inch chunk of ginger or 1 tbsp of ginger powder
½ a habanero or other hot pepper (optional)
1 tbsp fresh or dried basil
1 tbsp of dark miso
2 tbsp of light miso
2 tbsp of olive or canola oil
Bragg™ or soy sauce- to your tastes

Chop the daylights out of the above ingredients and place in a soup pot. Add the oil. Sauté until the mixture becomes semi-transparent. Add 6 cups of water. Bring to a boil. Turn on low and add the miso and Bragg™ or soy sauce. Simmer on low for 15 minutes. Add more or less water and miso depending on your tastes. Serves 2 to 3.

SOUP VARIATIONS:

Hearty Vegetable: Start with the soup base. Add any vegetables that you like. Some suggestions include carrots, spinach, collard greens, brussel sprouts, green onions and mushrooms. Add ½ cup of brown rice. Simmer on low for 45 minutes.

Tomato Dill: Start with the soup base. Add any veggies, such as carrots, broccoli, and spinach. Chop up some fresh dill—start with 2 tbsp and add more to your liking. Add crushed red chiles if you like spice. Add a 15 oz. can of tomato sauce. Simmer on low for 20 minutes.

Coconut Ginger: Start with the soup base, but double up on the fresh ginger. Add any veggies that you want. Add a 15 oz. can of coconut milk. Simmer on low for 20 minutes. Serve with brown rice.

Corn Chowder: Start with the soup base, but only use 4 cups of water. Add 2 bags of frozen corn. Simmer on low for 10 minutes. Place soup in a food processor or blender. Puree until creamy, adding water to obtain your desired consistency. Add salt and pepper to taste.

Minestrone: Start with the soup base. Add 1 can of plum tomatoes with the juice. Add thyme, rosemary, red pepper flakes, and extra basil. Dice 1 potato, 1 zucchini and 2 carrots and add to the soup. Add a ¼ cup of small pasta, your choice. Add ½ can of chickpeas. Cover and simmer for 15 minutes.

MEXICALI CHILI

Ingredients:
2 cans of pinto beans
1 can of black beans
1 can of kidney beans
1 can of diced tomatoes with juice
1 package of tempeh
3 cloves of garlic or 2 tbsp of garlic powder
1 bell pepper
1 medium onion
2 stalks of celery
1 jalapeno or habanero (optional)
2 tbsp fresh chopped cilantro (chopped)
1 tsp chili powder
1 tsp cumin
2 tbsp Bragg™ or soy sauce
2 tbsp apple cider vinegar or red wine vinegar
2 tbsp canola or olive oil
Soy cheese (optional)

Chop the onion, garlic and peppers. Combine oil, onion, garlic, and peppers in a soup pot and sauté on high for 3 minutes. Dice the tempeh into ¼ inch cubes and the celery into ½ inch slices. Add the remaining ingredients to the pot and add water to achieve desired consistency. Bring to a near boil, turn down heat, cover and simmer on low for 20 minutes. Top with shredded soy cheese and/or green onions. Serve with fresh bread or tortillas.

LASAGNA

Ingredients:
1 12 oz. package of oven ready lasagna noodles
1 medium size onion
1 bundle of fresh spinach
1 carton of mushrooms- any variety
1 zucchini
2 Tbsp olive oil
3 garlic cloves
4 tbsp of fresh basil or 2 tbsp of dried basil
2 15 oz. cans of tomato sauce or pizza sauce
1 package of firm tofu or vegan mozzarella
1 Tbsp red chili flakes (optional)
Nutritional Yeast to sprinkle on top

Chop the onions, garlic and basil and sauté in oil for 5 minutes on medium heat. Slice the mushrooms and zucchini and add to the sauté, adding water to keep moist. If using tofu, crumble the tofu and add to the sauté. Cook for five minutes on medium, add the spinach, cover and reduce heat. If using vegan mozzarella, grate or chop finely.

In a lightly-oiled baking pan, spread the tomato sauce on the bottom and then add one layer of the lasagna noodles. Add ½ of the sauté mixture and the vegan cheese, and add more tomato sauce on top. Add another layer of noodles, then the rest of the sauté mixture and vegan cheese and then more tomato sauce. Finish with another layer of noodles and cover with the remaining tomato sauce. Cover pan with foil and bake in a preheated 375°F oven for 40 minutes. Remove foil and bake for another 5-10 minutes to give the top layer a golden brown look. Sprinkle nutritional yeast on top and serve to your dearest family and friends.

TEMPEH TACOS

Ingredients:
1 package of tempeh
1 medium onion
3 cloves garlic or 1 tbsp of garlic powder
1 bell pepper
1 hot pepper (optional)
2 tbsp Bragg™ or soy sauce
2 tbsp canola or olive oil
Tortillas: corn or wheat
Optional condiments: pinto beans, shredded
lettuce, tomatoes, jalapenos and cilantro

Shred the tempeh with a food processor or cheese grater, or just chop until it has a ground beef consistency. Finely chop onion, garlic and peppers and combine with oil in a skillet. Sauté on high for 3 minutes or until onions begin to carmelize. Add the tempeh and Bragg™ and simmer on low for 10 minutes. Add water to keep the mixture moist. Warm the corn or flour tortillas. Roll the tempeh mixture in the tortillas with any condiments that you like.

STUFFED BELL PEPPERS

Ingredients:
4-6 big bell peppers, any color
1 15 oz. can of tomato sauce
1 medium sized onion
½ pound of mushrooms, any kind
1 bunch of fresh spinach
2 cloves garlic or 1 tbsp garlic powder
2 tbsp fresh or dried basil
1 hot pepper (optional)
1 cup cooked brown rice
¼ cup tempeh or vegan sausage (optional)
Bragg™ or soy sauce to taste

Chop all the ingredients except the bell peppers. In a skillet, add the oil, garlic, basil, hot pepper and onions and sauté on high for three minutes. Add the mushrooms and tempeh or sausage, and simmer on medium for 5 minutes. Add the spinach and rice, cover, and turn off heat.

Carefully cut the tops off the peppers, and place to the side. With a spoon, or your fingers, scoop out the seeds from the inside of the peppers. Fill the peppers with the sauté mixture and place the tops back on. Place peppers in a lightly oiled casserole dish and place in a preheated 350° oven. Bake until peppers are soft, usually 15 minutes. You can stuff the peppers with anything—try using the tempeh taco mixture, or create your own stuffing.

TERIYAKI TEMPEH

Ingredients:
1 package of tempeh
½ cup soy sauce or tamari
1 cup water
1 cloves garlic or 1 tbsp of garlic powder
1 inch chunk of ginger or 1 tbsp dried ginger
3 tbsp brown sugar
1 tsp sesame oil
2 tbsp corn starch or arrowroot

Combine the soy sauce, water, garlic, ginger and sugar in a sauce pan and bring to a boil. Lower heat to a low setting. Dissolve the corn starch in ¼ cup cold water and slowly add to the sauce, stirring constantly. If you want the sauce to be thicker, dissolve more corn starch or arrowroot in cold water and add to sauce. Cover and turn off heat. Slice the tempeh into ¼ inch cutlet strips. Place the oil and tempeh in a skillet over medium heat. Cook both sides until brown. You can also add vegetables such as broccoli and carrots to the dish.

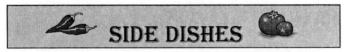

SIDE DISHES

OVEN FRIES

Ingredients:
Potatoes: any kind, including sweet potatoes
Olive or canola oil
salt to taste

Preheat oven to 450°F. Slice potatoes into ¼ slices. Lightly oil both sides and place on a baking sheet. Bake for 10 minutes and flip potatoes over. Bake until lightly browned.

MACARONI & "CHEESE"

Ingredients:
1 package of macaroni noodles
1 package of vegan soy cheese, cheddar flavor
¼ cup soy or rice milk
1 tsp canola or olive oil
salt to taste

Make pasta according to directions and drain. In a saucepan, combine the oil, milk, and cheese. Heat on medium, stirring often, until cheese melts. Pour over pasta and serve immediately.

HOMMUS AND BEAN DIPS

Ingredients:
2 cans of ready-to-eat garbanzo beans (chickpeas)
2 tbsp tahini
1 tbsp olive oil
1 clove of garlic
1 lemon, juiced
1 tbsp apple cider vinegar

Combine all the ingredients in a food processor. Puree until creamy, adding water until your desired consistency is achieved. Variations include adding roasted garlic, red peppers, olives, or sun-dried tomatoes. You can also add a shot of Bragg™ or soy sauce for additional flavor. For bean dips, substitute any beans that you like in place of the chickpeas. You can use pinto, black, red, kidney, and fava beans, just to name a few. Add cilantro and jalapenos if you desire.

GARLIC ROASTED POTATOES

Ingredients:
4 lbs of potatoes: any kind such as russets, red or
   Yukon gold
3 garlic cloves or 1 tbsp garlic powder
¼ cup olive oil
salt to taste

Finely chop the garlic. Cut the potatoes into ¼ inch spears (lengthwise). In a bowl, mix the garlic and oil thoroughly. Add the potatoes and toss well. Place the potatoes on a baking sheet in a 375°F preheated oven. Bake for about 40 minutes, turning potatoes over every 10 minutes.

MASHED POTATOES

Ingredients:
4 lbs of potatoes, russets or Yukon gold
2/3 cup of soy or rice milk
1 garlic clove or 1 tsp garlic powder
1 tsp canola or olive oil
salt to taste

Peel the potatoes and cut into cubes. Cook the potatoes in boiling water for 20 minutes or until soft. Drain and place in a bowl. Add the remaining ingredients and mash with a fork, potato masher or food processor adding water until desired consistency is achieved. Add salt to taste. Variations include adding roasted garlic and/or hot peppers. For curried mashed potatoes, simply add 1 tbsp of curry powder. You can also serve with a vegan gravy.

HASH BROWNS

Ingredients:
3 russet potatoes
1 medium sized onion, finely chopped
2 cloves garlic, finely chopped (optional)
2 tbsp canola oil
salt and pepper

Put potatoes in a pot of water and bring to a boil. Cook for 10 minutes or until half done. Take potatoes out of the water and allow to cool. When potatoes are cool enough to handle, remove the skin or leave it on. Grate the potatoes or just slice them into thin layers. Add the oil to a skillet or frying pan and heat under medium heat.

Add the onions and garlic in an even layer on the bottom of the pan. Add the potatoes in an even layer on top of the onions. Cook the potatoes undisturbed for 5-10 minutes or until the onions have started to carmelize. Carefully turn the mixture over. Cook the potatoes for an additional 5-10 minutes or until they turn brown. Add salt and pepper to taste. For a twist, add some grated tempeh to the mixture.

PANCAKES

Ingredients:
1 cup unbleached white flour
2 tbsp baking powder
1 tbsp raw cane sugar or sucanat
1 pinch of salt
1 cup soy milk
2 tbsp canola oil

Combine the dry ingredients in a bowl and mix thoroughly. Combine the wet ingredients in a separate bowl and mix thoroughly. Add the wet ingredients to the bowl with the dry ingredients and mix until a smooth batter. Pour onto a hot oiled griddle. When bubbles appear on the pancake, flip it and cook for another minute or two. This recipe makes 4 large sized pancakes. You can also use buckwheat or whole wheat flour. Variations include adding fresh berries, cooked apples, or vegan chocolate chips to the batter.

FRENCH TOAST

Ingredients:
3 ripe bananas
6 slice of bread- whole wheat works best
1 cup soy milk
2 tsp canola oil
2 tbsp maple syrup
¼ tsp cinnamon (optional)

Mash bananas in a bowl. Add the soy milk, maple syrup and cinnamon and mix well. Add the oil to a skillet or frying pan and heat under medium heat. Soak the bread slices in the mixture. Place in pan and lightly brown both sides.

BLUEBERRY MUFFINS

Ingredients:
2 cups unbleached white flour
¼ cup soy margarine or canola oil
½ cup applesauce or apple juice
1 cup sucanat or unrefined sugar
½ cup soymilk
1 tbsp baking powder
1 tsp vanilla
½ tsp salt
2 cups blueberries- fresh or frozen

Combine dry ingredients in a bowl and mix thoroughly. Combine wet ingredients in a separate bowl and mix thoroughly. Pour wet ingredients slowly into the bowl with the dry ingredients and mix until a smooth batter. Add the blueberries and mix well. Preheat oven to 350°F. Spray muffin cups with a nonstick spray. Fill cups ¾ full. Bake for 35 minutes or until tops are firm.

There are many variations to this recipe. You can use 1 cup of white flour and 1 cup of corn meal to make corn muffins. You can use whole wheat flour. You can add cinnamon and nutmeg. You can add vegan chocolate or carob chips. Experiment with all different flavors or make your own variety.

HANGOVER HELPER
(GREASY SPOON FEAST)

It is the morning after. You roll out of bed, the walls are spinning, the dog is barking way too loud.... make it to the couch. When you have had coffee, make this feast, you will feel much better. This has been a crowd pleaser for years. The recipe is a general guideline, tweak it anyway that you see fit.

> **Ingredients:**
> 3 russet potatoes
> 1 medium sized onion
> 1 bell pepper
> ½ package of Lightlife GimmeLean® Sausage
> ½ package of firm tofu (optional)
> 1 habanero or jalapeno pepper (optional)
> 3 cloves garlic or 2 tbsp garlic powder
> 3 tbsp olive or canola oil
> Bragg™ or soy sauce to taste
> kitchen sink (optional)

Chop the onion, garlic, and peppers. Cut the potatoes into cubes. Crumble the tofu. Grab a wok or a big pan. Add the onions, garlic, peppers, olive oil and Bragg™, and sauté for 5 minutes or until the onions begin to carmelize. Add the potatoes and sauté for 5 minutes on high, adding water as needed. Add the remaining ingredients, cover and simmer on low for 15 minutes.

The sausage comes in various shapes and sizes. If you buy the kind that comes in a tube-shaped package, slice the sausage into ¼ inch thick patties. In a lightly oiled skillet, cook the sausage until brown on both sides. If you like spice, add Tabasco™ or other hot sauce. Serve with toast, tortillas or a bagel.

CHOCOLATE MOUSSE CAKE

Ingredients:
1 cup couscous
2 ½ cups water
1 ½ cups sucanat or unrefined sugar
1 tbsp vanilla
¼ cup cocoa
1 10 oz. package Tropical Source™ chocolate chips
1 16 oz. package of firm tofu
3 tbsp maple syrup

In a saucepan, combine water, couscous, sucanat and cocoa. Bring to a simmer, stirring occasionally and cook until thickened (10 to 15 minutes). Add vanilla and stir. Spread mixture into a 9-inch spring form pan.

In a separate saucepan, melt chocolate chips **slowly** over low heat, stirring constantly. Transfer to a blender, add tofu and maple syrup and blend until smooth. Pour mixture over the couscous mixture and chill for at least an hour.

For a variation, you can spread toasted pecans on top of the couscous mixture before pouring the chocolate layer. You can also top the dessert with strawberries or raspberries.

Yum Yum Yum   Have FUN!

Appendix 2

NUTRIENT COMPARISONS OF FOOD ITEMS

Food Item	Serving Size	Protein (g)	Fat (g)	Calcium (mg)	Cholest. (mg)
Avocado	1 oz.	.6	2.8	3	0
Bagel	1 bagel	9.4	1.4	66	0
Banana	1 banana	1.3	.4	6	0
Beans, pinto	1 cup	15.4	1.1	79	0
Beef, ground	3 oz.	22.0	13.2	15	77
Beef, sirloin	3 oz.	22.9	12.1	17	64
Broccoli	1 cup	2.5	.3	41	0
Brussel sprouts	1 cup	3.9	.8	46	0
Butter	1 tbsp	.1	11.5	3	31
Carrots	1 cup	1.0	.3	36	0
Cheese, cheddar	1 oz.	7.1	9.4	204	30
Cheese, cottage	1 cup	28.0	2.3	156	18
Cheese, ricotta	1 cup	27.7	31.9	509	125
Chicken breast	½ breast	26.6	3.1	28	119
Chickpeas	1 cup	14.5	4.3	77	0
Collard Greens	1 cup	5.0	.7	357	0
Crab, Alaska	3 oz.	16.4	1.3	50	17
Lobster	3 oz.	17.4	.5	52	61
Shrimp	3 oz.	19.6	1.7	50	147
Egg	1 large	6.3	5.0	27	212
Cheeseburger	1 sandwich	28.2	32.9	206	88
Hot Dog	1 sandwich	10.4	14.5	24	44
Fish, cod	3 oz.	19.3	.7	18	40
Fish, halibut	3 oz.	22.7	2.5	51	35
Fish, salmon	3 oz.	16.8	5.1	181	47
Fish, swordfish	3 oz.	21.6	4.4	5	43
Fish, tuna	3 oz.	20.1	2.5	12	26
Ham	2 slices	9.4	4.9	14	32
Kale	1 cup	2.5	.5	179	0
Milk, whole	1 cup	7.9	7.9	276	24
Nuts, almonds	1 oz.	6.0	14.4	70	0
Peanuts	1 oz	7.9	14.0	15	0
Pork Chop	3 oz.	24.4	11.1	28	78
Rice, brown	1 cup	5.0	1.7	20	0
Soymilk	1 cup	10.9	4.7	93	0
Spinach	1 cup	7.6	.5	291	0
Turkey	3 oz	25.1	6.0	35	71
Termites	**100g**	**14.2**	**0**	**0**	**n/a**
Cap'n Crunch®	**¾ cup**	**1.1**	**1.6**	**4**	**0**

Appendix 3
VITAMINS

Vitamin	Vegan Sources	Good For
Vitamin A (Retinol or Beta-carotene)	carrots, leafy green vegetables, mangos, apricots, grapefruit	-bone development -immune system -eyesight
Vitamin B1 (Thiamin)	whole meal grains, sesame seeds, legumes, melons, peanuts	-converts glucose into energy -development of red blood cells
Vitamin B2 (Riboflavin)	leafy green vegetables, grains, legumes, avocados, mushrooms	-energy metabolism -eyesight -skin health
Vitamin B3 (Niacin)	whole meal grains, nuts, leafy green vegetables, sesame seeds, soy products	-metabolism -skin health -nervous and digestive systems
Vitamin B6 (Pyridoxine)	leafy green vegetables, whole meal grains, nuts, fruits	-metabolizing proteins -development of red blood cells -brain functioning -immune system
Vitamin B9 (Folate)	leafy green vegetables, legumes, seeds, citrus fruits	-development of red blood cells -assists in DNA synthesis
Vitamin B12 (Cyanocobalamin)	nutritional yeast, fortified soy products, supplements	-cell function -nervous system function
Vitamin C (Ascorbic Acid)	leafy green vegetables, citrus fruits, berries, cabbage, cauliflower. peppers, tomatoes	-healing of wounds -immune system -development of red blood cells
Vitamin D (Calciferol)	sunlight, fortified foods	-bone formation
Vitamin E (Tocopherol)	vegetable oils, vegetables, avocados, seeds and nuts	-antioxidant -development of red blood cells
Vitamin H (Biotin)	nuts, bananas, yeast	-synthesis and oxidation of fatty acids -helps utilize proteins
Vitamin K (Phylochinon)	broccoli, lettuce, cabbage, spinach, lentils	-essential for blood clotting -bone building

MINERALS

Mineral	Vegan Sources	Good For
Magnesium	leafy green vegetables, nuts	-bone development -nerves and muscles -metabolism and enzyme function
Phosphorous	nuts, whole meal grains, yeast extracts	-building teeth and bones -metabolic control
Iodine	sea vegetables, sea salt, iodized table salt, vegetables	-formation of hormones -health of skin, hair and nails
Iron	seeds, molasses, tofu, quinoa, oats, wheat, potatoes, ginger root, beans, sea vegetables	-healthy blood -immune system
Selenium	brazil nuts, molasses, sunflower seeds, whole grains, oatmeal	-enzyme production -immune system -eradication of free radicals
Zinc	seeds, nuts, wheat, quinoa, oats, beans	-immune function -reproduction -respiration -wound healing -growth and development

Appendix 4

FOOD ADDITIVES

This appendix lists some common food additives that are derived from animal products. This list is by no means exhaustive as there are many food ingredients.

Food Additive	What is It
Albumen	Usually derived from eggs
Casein and Caseinates	Milk protein
Chitin	Produced from crab & shrimp shells
Cochineal	Made from crushed insects
Gelatin	Made from the bones, skins, hoofs, and tendons of cows, pigs, fish and other animals.
Lactates, Lactic acid, Lactose	Milk protein
Lecithin	Usually made from soy beans, but can be made from eggs
Monoglycerides and Diglycerides	Made from animal fat
Pepsin	Enzyme derived from a pig's stomach
Stearic Acid and Stearates	Derived from animal fat
Whey	Byproduct of cheese making
Worcester Sauce- used in most Bloody Mary mixes	Contains anchovies

Appendix 5

VARIOUS RESEARCH STUDIES

The British Medical Association

Vegetarians have lower rates of obesity, coronary heart disease, high blood pressure, large bowel disorders, cancers and gall stones. Vegetarians are about 40 percent less likely to get cancer than non-vegetarians, regardless of other risks such as smoking. Vegetarians obtain all the minerals they need, folate levels are higher and as a consequence it is a diet suitable for infants.

The China Health Study

This study looked at the health and eating habits of 6,500 Chinese people. It found that the greatest single influence on the growth of diseases such as heart disease, cancer, strokes and diabetes was the amount of animal fat and animal protein eaten. The more one eats, the greater the risk. The study also found that meat was not the best source of iron. The Chinese diet was predominantly vegetarian and yet adults consumed twice as much iron as an American adult.

The World Health Organization

This study found that a diet high in animal products promotes heart disease, cancer and several other diseases. It confirmed the BMA's and China Health Study's list of diseases and added osteoporosis and kidney failure as being related to meat eating. In 2003, there was an updated study which reaffirmed the original, stating that the worldwide dietary trend towards high saturated fat and refined carbohydrate foods, together with sedentary lifestyles are the principal causes of degenerative diseases.

The EPIC Study

In 1993 the largest study of diet and health was initiated—the European Prospective Investigation into Cancer and Nutrition (EPIC). More than half a million people were studied in ten European countries. EPIC studies have confirmed the importance of a diet rich in fruits and vegetables as protection against the risk of an early death. Frequent consumption of red meat is associated with a 20-40% increase in colon cancer risk. Vegetarian diets reduce blood pressure levels, cholesterol levels and obesity.

Physicians Committee for Responsible Medicine (PCRM)

In 1995 the PCRM, an organization of more than 5,000 doctors and scientists, issued a report to the U.S. Government. It urged the government to recommend a vegetarian diet to U.S. citizens. Until then, the U.S. Dietary Guidelines had never made any mention of vegetarianism. The following year they did so for the first time:

> "...vegetarians enjoy excellent health: Vegetarian diets are consistent with Dietary Guidelines and can meet the Recommended Daily Allowances for nutrients. Protein is not limited in vegetarian diets ..."

American Dietetic Association (ADA)

The ADA issued a report on vegetarianism, saying it is effective in avoiding and curing some of the world's most deadly diseases. According to the ADA, heart disease, strokes, some cancers and diabetes can all be largely prevented by adhering to a vegetarian diet. Vegetarian diets can provide all the vitamins, minerals, protein and energy that the body needs and provide for all stages of life including pregnancy and infancy.

Appendix 6

SOURCES

Websites:

www.vegetarian.org.uk: Vegetarian & Vegan Foundation. *"Safeguarding Children's Health"*, *"Your Health in Your Hands."*

www.eatveg.com: "The Average American Eats in a Lifetime."

www.beyondveg.com: Billings, Tom *"Paleodiet and Paleolithic Nutrition."*

www.janegoodall.com: The Jane Goodall Institute. *"Hunting."*

www.onelife.com: Stevenson, John. *"The Evolution of Man."*

www.geocities.com/Heartland/Cottage/1288/intro/Intro.htm: "Introduction to Cheesemaking."

www.whymilk.com: the online educational resource for consumers from MilkPep, (Milk Processors Education Program), funded by America's Milk Processors. *"Fuel for Athletes"*

www.asiarecipe.com/burgypsy.html: "Sea Gypsy: The Salon People of Myanmar", 2005.

www.fieldandstream.com: Herring, Hal, *"Don't Eat That Fish"*, Field and Stream,. 2005.

www.vnv.org.au: Ogilvie, David, *"So What's Wrong With Fishing"*, Vegetarian Network Victoria.

www.vegansociety.com: "Beer and Wine", 2005.

www.cspinet.org/reports/chemcuisine.htm: "Food Safety Food Additives" , May 25, 2005.

www.americanheart.org: American Heart Association. *"Trans Fatty Acids"*, *"Fat Substitutes"*, *"Fish and Omega-3 Fatty Acids"*, August, 2005.

www.hormel.com: "Canned Products"

www.bragg.com: "Liquid Aminos Info", 2005.

U.S. Government Research:

United States Department of Agriculture. *"America's Eating Habits: Changes and Consequences"*, USDA Economic Research Service, Food and Rural Economics Division: Agriculture Information Bulletin No. 750, February, 2000.

United States Department of Agriculture. *"Testimony of Eric M. Bost Under Secretary, Food, Nutrition and Consumer Services Before the House Committee on Government Reform Subcommittee on Human Rights and Wellness,"* September 15, 2004.

United States Department of Agriculture. *"USDA National Nutrient Database for Standard Reference, Release 17"*.

National Academy of Sciences. *"Dietary Reference Intakes"*, 2004.

U.S. Department of Health and Human Services and U.S. Environmental Protection Agency. *"Public Health Implications of Exposure to Polychlorinated Biphenyls (PCBs)"*, 2005.

U.S. Department of Health and Human Services and U.S. Environmental Protection Agency. *"What You Need To Know About Mercury in Fish and Shellfish"*, March 2004.

U.S. Food and Drug Administration. *"Food Allergies Rare But Risky"*, FDA Consumer, May 1994: Updated December 2004.

United States Department of Agriculture. *"Dietary Guidelines for Americans 2005- Appendix B"*.

United States Department of Agriculture. *"Organic Food Standards and Labels: The Facts"*, April 2002.

US Food and Drug Administration & International Food Information Council Foundation. *"Food Ingredients & Colors"*, November, 2004.

Executive Office of The President, Office of Management and Budget. *"To Save Lives, OMB Urges Revising Dietary Guidelines"*, May 28, 2003.

United States Department of Agriculture. *"US Dietary Guidelines"*, federal advisory committees nutritional recommendations to Secretaries of Agriculture, Health and Human Services, 1995, p.21.

United States Department of Agriculture, The National Organic Program *"Organic Food Standards and Labels: The Facts"*, April 2002.

Foulke, Judith E., U.S. Food and Drug Administration, *"A Fresh Look at Food Preservatives"*, FDA Consumer, October 1993.

130

Segal, Marian, U.S. Food and Drug Administration, *"Fat Substitutes: A Taste of the Future?"*, FDA Consumer, December 1990.

Independent Research:

Harvard School of Public Health. *"Fruits and Vegetables"*, *<http://www.hsph.harvard.edu/nutritionsource/fruits.html>*, (August 1, 2005).

Nieman, David C. *"Physical fitness and vegetarian diets: is there a relation?"*, Am J Clin Nutr 1999;70(suppl):570S-5S.

Forbes-Ewan, Chris. *"Effect of Vegetarian Diets on Performance in Strength Sports"*, *<http://www.sportsci.org/jour/0201/cf-e.htm>*, (June 5, 2005).

Kleiner, Susan M Phd. *"The Role of Meat in an Athlete's Diet: It's Effect on Key Macro-nutrients"*, SSE#58, Volume 9 (1995), Number 5.

World Health Organization. *"Diet, Nutrition and the prevention of Chronic Diseases"* 1991. Technical Report Series 797.

American Dietetic Association. *"Vegetarian Diets"*, <http://www.eatright.org/Member/PolicyInitiatives/index_21026.cfm.> (August 11, 2005).

Physicians Committee for Responsible Medicine. *"The Protein Myth"*, *<http://www.pcrm.org/health/veginfo/protein.html>*, (July 20, 2005).

National Cancer Institute. *"Heterocyclic Amines in Cooked Meats"*, September 15, 2004.

Willett, W.C. *"Micronutrients and cancer risk"*. AJCN;59(Suppl.):1162S-1165S, 1994.

Curhan, G.C. et al., *"A prospective study of dietary calcium and other nutrients and the risk of symptomatic kidney stones"*., NEJM;328:833-838, 1993.

American Heart Association. *"Heart Attack and Angina Statistics"*, Oct. 3, 2003.

M. Thorogood et al. *"Plasma Lipids and Lipoproteins in Groups With Different Dietary Practices Within Britain,"* British Medical Journal 295 (1987): 351-3.

Ornish, Dean et al. *"Intensive lifestyle changes for reversal of coronary heart disease"*, JAMA;280(23):2001-2007, 1998.

Harvard School of Public Health. *"Calcium & Milk"*, 2004.

44

Feskanich D, Willett W.C., Stampfer M.J., Colditz G.A. *"Milk, dietary calcium, and bone fractures in women: a 12-year prospective study"*. *Am J Public Health* 1997; 87:992-7.

Owusu et al. *"Calcium Intake and the Incidence of Forearm and Hip Fractures among Men"*, Journal of Nutrition Vol. 127 No. 9 Septemebr 1997 pp 1782-1787.

Cumming R.G., Klineberg R.J. *"Case-control study of risk factors for hip fractures in the elderly."* Am J Epidemiol 1994;139:493-505.

Ornish D., Brown S.E., Scherwitz L.W., Billings J.H., Armstrong W.T., Ports T.A. *"Can lifestyle changes reverse coronary heart disease?"* Lancet 1990;336:129-33.

Scott F.W. *"Cow milk and insulin-dependent diabetes mellitus: is there a relationship?"*, Am J Clin Nutr 1990;51:489-91.

Karjalainen J, Martin JM, Knip M, et al. *"A bovine albumin peptide as a possible trigger of insulin-dependent diabetes mellitus."* N Engl J Med 1992;327:302-7.

Bertron P, Barnard ND, Mills M. *"Racial bias in federal nutrition policy, part I: the public health implications of variations in lactase persistence"*. J Natl Med Assoc 1999;91:151-7.

Srinivasan R and Minocha A. *"When to suspect lactose intolerance: symptomatic, ethnic and laboratory clues"*, Postgrad. Med., 1999; 104(3):pp.109-123.

Goulding, et al, *"Children Who Avoid Drinking Cow's Milk Are at Increased Risk for Prepubertal Bone Fractures"*, Journal of the American Dietetic Association, 2004.

Matkovic, et al. *"Nutrition Influences Skeletal Development from Childhood to Adulthood: a Study of Hip, Spine, and Forearm in Adolescent Females"*, J Am Diet Assoc. 2004.

Kalkwarf, et al, *"Milk intake during childhood and adolescence, adult bone density, and osteoporotic fractures in U.S. Women."* Am J CLin Nutr 2003; 77:257-65.

Hightower, Jane and Moore, Dan. *"Mercury Levels in High-end Consumers of Fish"*, Environmental Health Perspectives, April 2003.

Environmental Defense. *"PCBs in Fish and Shellfish"*, August 29, 2004.

People for the Ethical Treatment of Animals. *"Think Fish is Health Food, Think Again"*, 2005.

132

Edwards, Rob. *"Farmed Salmon more contaminated than wild"*, NewScientist.com, January 9, 2004.

Weiss, Kenneth R. *"Fish Farms Become Feedlots of the Sea"*, LA Times, December 9, 2002.

Pyevich, Caroline. *"Why is Wine so Fined?"*, Vegetarian Journal, 1997.

United States Sugar Corporation. *"Sugar Refining"*, *<http://www.ussugar.com/sugar/sugar%20refining.html>*, (May 25, 2005).

National Honey Board. *"Honey and Antioxidants"*, *<http://www.nhb.org/nutrition/nutritionResearch.html>*, (May 25 2005).

University of Maryland Medical Center. *"Blood Diseases: Iron-Deficiency Anemia"*, 2005.

Mangels, Reed P.H.D., *<http://www.vrg.org/nutrition/iron.htm>* , *"Iron in the Vegan Diet"*.

Larsson, Christel L and Johansson, Gunnar K. *"Dietary intake and nutritional status of young vegans and omnivores in Sweden"*, 2002.

Ball, Madeleine J, Bartlett, Melinda A. *"Dietary intake and iron status of Australian vegetarian women"*, Am J Clin Nutr 1990, 70:353-8, 1999.

Wilson A.K., Ball, M.J. School of Nutrition and Public Health, *"Nutrient intake and iron status of Australian male vegetarians"*, Deakin University, Melbourne, Australia, Eur J Clin Nutr. 1999 Mar;53(3):189-94.

Hunt, Janet R, *"Bioavailability of iron, zinc, and other trace minerals from vegetarian diets."* Am J Clin Nutr 2003, 78(suppl).

Craig, W.J. *"Iron status of vegetarians"*, Department of Nutrition, Andrews University, Berrien Springs, MI. Am J Clin Nutr. 1994 May;59(5 Suppl):1233S-1237S.

Harman, S.K., Parnell, W.R. *"The nutritional health of New Zealand vegetarian and non-vegetarian Seventh-day Adventists selected vitamin, mineral and lipid levels."*, Department of Human Nutrition, university of Otago, Dunedin. N Z Med J. 1998 Mar 27;111(1062).

Larsson, Christel L and Johansson, Gunnar K. *"Dietary intake and nutritional status of young vegans and omnivores in Sweden"*, 2002.

Messina, Virginia, MPH, RD, Messina, Mark, PhD , *"The Vegetarian Way: Total Health for You and Your Family"* (1996), p. 102.

Parnell, Harman S.K. *"The nutritional health of New Zealand vegetarian and non-vegetarian Seventh-day Adventists: selected vitamin, mineral and lipid levels"*, N Z Med J. 1998 Mar 27;111(1062):91-4.

133

Harvard School of Public Health, *"Vitamins"*, <*http://www.hsph.harvard.edu/nutritionsource/vitamins.html*>, (May 26, 2005).

Craig, Alsion. Pesticide Action Network UK. *"People's Pesticide Exposure: Poisons we are exposed to everyday without knowing it"*, December 2004.

Consumers Union. *"Press Release"*, February 18, 1999.

Institute of Food Science & Technology. *"ISFT: Current Hot Topics- Organic Food"*, February, 2005.

Worthington, Virginia. "*Nutritional Quality of Organic Versus Conventional Fruits, Vegetables, and Grains*," The Journal of Alternative and Complementary Medicine, Vol. 7, No. 2, 2001 (pp. 161-173).

Avery, Alex A. *"The Deadly Chemicals in Organic Food"*, Hudson Institute March 28, 2002.

British Medical Association. *"Genetically modified foods and health: a second interim statement"* , March 2004, page 3.

The Glutomate Association. *"MSGFacts"*, <http://www.msgfacts.com/facts/msgfacts.html>, (May 25, 2005).

Farlow, Dr. Christine. *"Poisons in Your Unborn Baby's Food"*, Healthy Eating Advisory, <*http://www.healthyeatingadvisor.com/foodadditives-unbornbabies.html*>, (May 25, 2005).

Blaylock, Dr. Russell, *"Hidden Sources of MSG in Foods"* from the book "Excitotoxins; The Taste That Kills", <http://www.rense.com/general52/msg.htm>, (May 25, 2005).

Institute of Medicine of the National Academies. *"Dietary Reference Intakes: Water, Potassium, Sodium, Chloride, and Sulfate."* February 11, 2004.

British Medical Association. *"Diet, Nutrition & Health"*, BMA Report, 4.11, p49 1986.

Cambell T C, et al. *"Study on Diet, Nutrition and Disease in the People's Republic of China"*, Cornell University, 1989.

World Health Organization. *"Diet, Nutrition and the prevention of Chronic Diseases"*, 1991. Technical Report Series 797.

134

Books:

Barnard, Neal. *"Food for Life"* (New York: Harmony Books, 1993), p. 34.

Pennington, J. *"Food Values of Portions Commonly Used"*, Harper and Row, 14th ed. New York, 1985.

Morgan, Elaine, *"The Aquatic Ape: A Theory of Human Evolution"*, Stein and Day, 1982.

Schiosser E. *"Fast Food Nation: The Dark Side of the All-American Meal"*, New York, NY: Houghton Mifflin, 2001.

Other:

Albert Einstein Archives. Letter to Hans Muehsam, March 30, 1954, AEA 38-435.

American Egg Board. *"Nutrition Label"* 2005.

Hostess® Twinkies® Ingredient label

Doctor Fun Cartoons (*http://www.ibiblio.org/Dave/drfun.htm*)

God. Exodus 3:8, Old Testament, B.C.